Robert Renn's Complete Book of Hair Coloring

Robert Renn's Complete Book of Hair Coloring

Illustrations by Martha Voutas

 Random House New York

All rights reserved under International and Pan-American Copyright Conventions.
Published in the United States by Random House, Inc., New York, and
simultaneously in Canada by Random House of Canada Limited, Toronto.

Photograph of Mary Randolph Carter Berg, *Mademoiselle*,
July 1977. Courtesy *Mademoiselle* magazine, Copyright
© 1977 by The Condé Nast Publications, Inc.

Library of Congress Cataloging in Publication Data
Renn, Robert, 1940-
Robert Renn's Complete book of hair coloring.
Includes index.
1. Hair—Dyeing and bleaching. I. Title.
II. Title: Complete book of hair coloring.
TT973.R46   646.7'243   79–4771
ISBN 0–394–50370–8

Manufactured in the United States of America

Design by Bernard Klein

98765432

First Edition

*Reports made by the National Cancer Institute in 1978
indicated that certain chemicals used in hair dyes caused cancer
in laboratory animals. None of the products recommended in my book
contain those chemicals, and many major hair-coloring manufacturers
have recently eliminated them from their permanent hair-coloring
formulas.*

ROBERT RENN

Acknowledgments

My sincerest thanks to Francesco Scavullo, who started the ball
rolling, for it was while I was working on his beauty book that I met
his editor, Susan Bolotin. She and Ellen Coughlin encouraged me to
write this book; I am deeply grateful to all three.

Much gratitude to Mallory Hathaway for help and assistance
when I needed it the most; to Joel Broadsky for his fine color
photographs; to Jackie Farber, my editor; to Martha Voutas, for her
illustrations; and to the production staff of Random House for their
design and for the finished book.

Thanks to my cover girl, Rene Russo, and to Way Bandy for her
exciting makeup.

And a most special thanks go to my assistants, Dale and Tom,
who, while enduring much hard work, have been so patient and
enthusiastic.

Contents

What
I Believe

There is nothing more striking nor more beautiful than healthy, glorious, natural-looking hair—hair as shining with highlights and lowlights as a child's—glinted and shaded with tones of the same value. This is the color I give to my clients. Such color does not come out of a bottle alone. It comes from an attitude about haircolor, which I would like to pass on to you. That attitude, or philosophy of hair coloring as I like to think of it, combined with the right coloring products, should give you the wherewithal for a glorious head of hair. With a minimum guide to a few select color methods and with a maximum look at taste, you can pull all your beauty features into focus. This is Robert Renn hair color.

Hair color can dramatically change your looks; only

expensive plastic surgery can do more. Hair color can achieve maximum effects for the least amount of time and money. When done correctly, color can warm up dull drab hair; it can cover gray; and it can make hair more shiny and alive. Color can give your hair new body and actually improve the condition and texture. Hair color can camouflage a facial fault. I believe that the proper hair color does more for the total person than any other beauty technique. If you look more beautiful on the outside—and you will with the right color—you will feel more beautiful on the inside.

With the hundreds of products on the market today, you could choose just the right color, or, more likely, be totally confused. This book will show you how to find the perfect hair color for you—color that will do the most for your features and your skin tone, that will not chain you to constant up keep, and that will use the least amount of chemicals. I have already done the experimenting for you. Nineteen years in the beauty business, as well as working for films, television and theater, and for top fashion magazines, have given me the knowledge to achieve just the right look with the least amount of effort and have brought me a select clientele, including some of the most famous people in the world.

Everyone has the right to look better and to be at her most beautiful. The right hair color can help you achieve your perfect look and I will show you how to find it, inexpensively and easily. After you've read this guide to color, you will have a working knowledge of the different color processes, and you will be able to give yourself at home, at just a drop of the cost, a custom-salon look. My methods and formulas have been carefully developed and simplified through years of experience and experimentation, and will give proper results without the chance of risk for you—results which, when done in good taste, would only be equaled by my doing the work in the salon.

Working on this project has been exciting. I started out expecting to express my ideas so that they could be of use to many people. But by breaking down and simplifying my methods, and by taking a much closer look at my work, I now have a new and refreshed concept of hair coloring. I knew from the start that my book would benefit all of you who would like to be guided in the use of hair color, but I didn't realize that the one person who would get the most out of it would be me.

Hair Color by Choice— Not by Chance

Though my intention is to teach you to color your hair at home, if you feel you must go to a professional you should know as much about hair color, as much about your particular needs in color and, most important, as much about your hair colorist as possible. The professional hair colorist has a serious responsibility—your color, your hair's condition, your total hair —and you deserve the best.

Before I do someone's hair for the first time, I ask her to see me first for a consultation. This enables me to decide what kind of color the client will need and exactly how much time will be needed for the first appointment. We talk about skin color to be sure the new hair color will be complementary, about price, and about the processes I will use—processes with little or no peroxide and which will require the least amount of maintenance. None of the products that I use in my salon, and none that I will recommend to you for use at home, contain any chemicals suspected of being carcinogenic.

Sometimes I consult with people who come to me for professional advice but who will listen only to what they want to hear. These are people who have pre-established ideas. One may be a brunette who has decided to go platinum blonde; another is unhappy with the way her hair is looking but is unwilling to change the process; a third may be someone whose hair is so damaged that it would be dangerous to work on it until conditioning and time would make it possible. These are the people who are impossible to please and who often will demand that I do something that I don't believe in. They really don't need me, and I recommend that they go somewhere else. I care about the way my clients' hair looks, just as any professional should.

Sometimes when people come to me for a consultation, I really can't believe what I'm seeing. I see olive complexions with flaming red hair; hair that has been so overfrosted that it looks gray; or platinum blondes who have an inch of dark at the roots. I'm glad they've come to me for help, but I'm amazed at how they got themselves into these situations in the first place.

You may, like a lot of people, think that fads are exciting and want to change your looks and hair color accordingly. Fads can be exciting, but only if they are appropriate to you and your lifestyle. A constant "trying-on" process will never work and can end up in disaster, damaging not only your hair but your sense of who you are. The person who knows who she is will naturally know how to be the most attractive. Taste and moderation always win out.

Most people think that looking well is only a matter of beauty and is not a question of self-respect, assurance and confidence. To be educated in how to get this kind of confidence at home and how to make the most of what you've got—whether you are male or female, young or old—is what beauty is all about. People who weren't born beautiful can learn to make themselves more exciting and more together, but beautiful people need a little help too.

Pick out elegant people on television or at a party and notice what they wear. You'll probably not see anything extreme and will see all aspects working together to achieve a total look. Notice how flamboyant are the hair styles or vivid hair colors worn by people who are basically not attractive. Why does a woman with the brightest red hair wear a vivid orange or shocking-colored dress? Good taste comes from simplicity and in knowing yourself. Do you get my message? Be yourself, work with what you have and find the hair colorist who agrees with this philosophy.

If you aren't going to do your own color at home, then it is vital that you learn not only how to find the right professional for you but how to communicate with him when you do find him. First, how do you find the right professional? In large cities the beauty business has been turning into a very specialized industry. Usually people who specialize in one area of the business, such as hair coloring, are more knowledgeable as well as more experienced than a person with a one-man full-service operation, who gives everything from permanents to pedicures. If your town does not have someone who specializes in color, find the person who has the most experience in hair coloring and interview *him*. If you see someone whose hair you really like, don't be embarrassed to stop her on the street or in a restaurant and ask who did her color. People always love to get compliments. You can bring in a photograph or drawing to illustrate what you'd like to try when you've found your colorist. Some professionals may turn up their noses at this, but I have found, whether or not the look is good for the individual, it is very helpful in giving me a direction for the client. Remember, telephone ahead to set up an appointment for a consultation before any work is done, and always make sure that all prices are discussed.

Above all, find a patient, professional hair colorist. In order to discuss all of your color problems and work out a new program—one which will not only correct the color but will eventually improve the condition and overall health of your hair —your colorist must be understanding. On the other hand, you too must be patient. If your hair is damaged, a good colorist will recommend conditioning treatments before any coloring is to be done. He also might suggest that you let your hair grow out a bit more, so that some of the damaged ends can be trimmed and so that the new healthy growth can then be color-treated. Make sure your professional has a sense of responsibility to your hair and to you, too.

I have found that most people come to me through personal recommendations. Models are sent to me by their agencies, some people hear about me from friends, and there are many who have come clutching magazine articles in their hands.

About 75 percent of the people I see for consultation need some kind of corrective hair coloring. Fifteen percent of the people I see for consultation have been coloring their hair but are either bored with their old color or feel trapped by a frequent maintenance program.

The final 10 percent of my new clients are those who have never colored their hair before. They range from young women who would like to do something to make themselves more exciting, to women who have just begun to go gray.

Whether you are going to do your hair at home or rely on a professional hair colorist, you must know your hair and your needs before you can start on any program, and this is what this book is all about. Hair color by choice—not by chance.

What You Must Know Before You Decide to Color

Once you've made the decision to color your hair at home, you will find that you are confronted with shelves of products, all promising wonderful results but all with different ways of achieving them. Now you have to make the decision as to whether you want a temporary rinse or a permanent bleach . . . you could buy a frosting kit . . . or what about shampoo-in color, or paint-on color, or brush-through color?

Keeping in mind that the wrong choice will be absolutely disastrous, this is the time to ask yourself the questions that I ask of everyone who comes to me.

1. What do you want hair coloring to do for you?
2. What kind of hair do you have?

3. What is the condition of your hair?
4. How much color maintenance can you afford in terms of both time and dollars?
5. What color will complement your skin tone?

You *can* achieve dramatic color effects at home—for under ten dollars you can have a professional look that would cost many times that in a salon. You can tailor hair coloring to fit your lifestyle—but your success will come from your answers to these questions before purchasing any one product.

I. What Will Hair Coloring Do for You?

Hair coloring does far more than transform a brunette into a blonde—and it rarely does that well. It should supply body, improve texture, brighten tones, give shine or camouflage gray or graying hair. I will guarantee you'll be disappointed if you are not honest with yourself about what you expect to achieve by changing the natural color of your hair. *Don't* expect to look like the model on the package, no matter how carefully you follow the instructions.

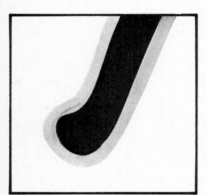

Color can: 1) add body

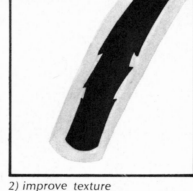

2) improve texture

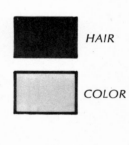

HAIR

COLOR

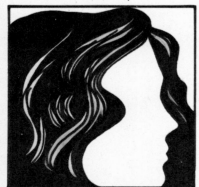

3) give shine

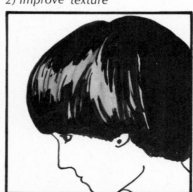

4) improve tone

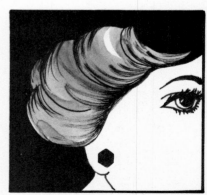

5) cover gray

2. What Kind of Hair Do You Have?

As you look at your hair, some adjectives come easily to mind—straight, wavy or curly. (Surprised?) Straight or fine hair will show the most subtle color changes and therefore makes coloring mistakes more obvious. Curly hair, though, can hide a multitude of coloring or cutting sins. And because it curls, the hair also hides new growth. Thus, curly heads can experiment with more exaggerated color effects.

TEXTURE

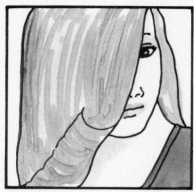

Straight

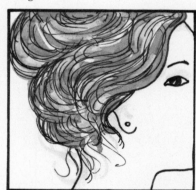

Fine

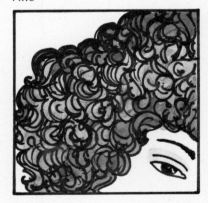

Curly

Hair is also classified as fine, medium or coarse. These terms describe *texture,* not *thickness.* Texture relates to the individual hair shaft, thickness to the density of hair on the head. Hair treatments such as coloring and permanent waves expand the hair shaft, changing the texture and giving added body, making each hair seem fatter.

A head of hair can be both fine and thick. Blacks, for instance, have curly hair that may look coarse because of its thickness but is actually fine and soft to the touch.

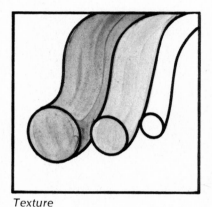

Texture

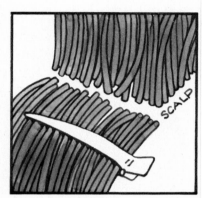

Density or Thickness

NOTE: Texture does not remain the same throughout your life. If you are turning gray, you will notice that new hair comes in coarser, almost wiry. You may also notice differences if you have had a recent operation or are taking medication, since your state of health affects hair. Some medications lengthen color-processing time, making results unpredictable. If you have any questions, check with your doctor before coloring.

Childbirth, too, can affect your hair. For three or four months afterward, hair often becomes dry and fragile, which sometimes results in hair loss. If you want a morale-booster, a change in hair color can do it. But condition carefully first, then choose a gentle coloring process. And don't forget the patch test. There'll be more about that later.

3. What Is the Condition of Your Hair?

Is your hair naturally dry or oily? Since coloring and permanents (or straightening) tend to dry the hair, anyone with hair on the dry side should keep coloring at a minimum. However, oily hair can profit from processing, as proper color can equalize the situation, giving hair more body as the oily condition seems to be corrected.

Is your hair damaged from overprocessing by other treatments or from overexposure to wind, sun or chlorine? Ends show wear and tear first, especially with long hair. If you have dry ends and want to color, remember to apply the treatment only to the main part of the hair, leaving the ends untouched until the last few minutes of processing, if you color them at all. I find that if the ends remain slightly lighter than the rest of the hair, the effect is softer and more natural anyway.

WARNING: The results of color will be only as good as the condition of your hair. Correct any problems before applying color treatments.

4. How Much Maintenance Can You Afford?

Don't be a slave to your roots. The more drastic the change in your natural hair color, the more you are chained to color processing. New hair grows on the average of one-fourth of an inch each month. A radical transformation from brunette to blonde would require constant maintenance. But sophisticated highlights can be achieved with far less time and trouble—and might need to be repeated only three or four times a year instead of every three or four weeks. I would never change a brunette to a blonde, unless of course it was for an actress who had to be transformed for a role.

5. What Color Will Complement Your Skin Tone?

Before you color your hair you must consider skin tone. It, rather than your natural or sought – after hair color, is what makes or breaks a new color look. And like hair texture, skin tone can change with age and from season to season. It is absolutely vital to be aware of your skin tone.

There are six basic skin tones: creamy white, pink, ruddy, sallow, olive and brown/black. To determine your true skin color, remove all makeup, put a white scarf or turban around your head and wear white or neutral-colored clothing. Stand in natural light—outdoors or at a window—and (this is the difficult part) look in the mirror. If you are still undecided after a look in the mirror under these conditions, ask two friends what they think. You get the idea? Only after deciding what your correct skin color is can you choose the best complementary hair color.

Creamy white skin tone is the old peaches-and-cream complexion. Almost all hair colors complement this skin tone and none clash. But dark or brunette colors tend to be more dramatic, supplying greater contrast. Pale-blond shades lack contrast and wash out the skin tone. Therefore blond shades should always be on the dark side if your skin is creamy white.

Pink skin tones can be toned down with proper makeup, but when coloring hair, avoid strawberry or red shades, which will only accent what you want to disguise. If your natural hair color is red, tone down to a darker auburn for a softer, more natural look. Remember: just because something *is* natural doesn't mean it *looks* natural. I recommend light toast brown or the ash shades in blond or brown for pink skin.

Ruddy skin tones are often associated with redheads and freckles, but if you have a heavy suntan or an outdoor look most of the year, you're probably ruddy-toned, too. Brassy tones should be played down because they match rather than contrast with this skin tone. Contrast your skin tone with darker or lighter shades. A ruddy skin tone could go blond for a surfer or Scandinavian multi-blond, but only if the color is sandy with a minimum of red and gold. Avoid solid dark color by softening with different tones of brown.

Light-olive or sallow skin tones go best with soft-brown hair coloring or with highlights of lighter, neutral-brown or soft-beige streaks. At all costs, avoid red or gold tones, which tend to make sallow skin look yellow.

Olive skin tones glow when hair coloring is warm brown, or dark and shining brunette complemented with subtle shadings. Colors of the same brown value or one or two tones lighter will also work. But beware of that red, henna-hussy look, which has been the rage in Europe. Red next to olive gives a green tinge to the skin, so olive skin only ends up looking sun-cooked, brittle and hard. Blondes might also have olive skin, but the new shade should be a definite no-red ash blond.

Brown/black skin tones, like olive, should avoid reds. A subtle contrast is most flattering—slightly darker hair on brown skins—slightly lighter on black. Very subtle shadings of brown on brown tones, or a combination of dark, earth tones would be perfect.

Now you're ready to take the plunge. I've outlined your hair-color needs and have matched your skin tone to your best complementary hair color. I've given you my basic pointers to make hair color work for you and you know what you should expect from proper hair coloring. My next step will be to show you how to choose the correct product and method to ensure your perfect color.

How to use the chart

By matching (as closely as possible) your natural hair color to one of those shown at the top of the chart, and reading straight down, you will be able to get the best results for your skin tone—all with a minimum of harsh chemicals and the least amount of maintenance.

1 NATURAL HAIR COLOR	**The old you**
2 SKIN TONE	**Your real skin tone without makeup**
3 PROBLEM AND SOLUTION	**What's wrong with your natural hair color and why does it not work for you?**
4 METHOD	1.) **Process—How to achieve results** 2.) **Maintenance—How often it must be done** 3.) **How to treat gray to achieve results**
	The Wonderful New You!

What Kind of Color to Buy and How to Use It at Home

There are many products on the market that you can buy in your drugstore or in beauty-supply houses. They are the products that you will use at home to get the look that most approximates what I would try to give you if you came to my salon. There are many different products, and although I am going to discuss all the different types, and even give you my special directions for using them, I really believe to get the most from your hair—to give it the healthy and glorious look that I feel is my trademark—there are only two processes that I can heartily recommend. The first is the single-process, new five-week rinse type (such as Revlon's Young Hair NCT and Clairol's Beautiful Browns), which I use in my salon as a replacement for the tints with peroxide. The second is a highlighting process which I have refined from the standard frosting kit. I am going to give you special directions for these processes, singling them out from the many others that I talk about. But since there are many products on the market, and since you might want a quickie touch-up or a color rinse at one time or another, I am going to talk about all the products available to you and tell you how to use them, offering special Renn Hints to refine and modify the directions. Are you ready?

Don't be confused by all the hair-color products you see on your drugstore or beauty supplier's shelves. All hair coloring falls into just three categories:

1. Temporary Color
2. Semi-Permanent Color
3. Permanent Color

I will be discussing the various processes that fall into these three categories, giving you examples of products in each instance. Remember, these products are not necessarily my recommendations, but are mentioned only to assist you in understanding the type of product used in each specific process. When I wish to recommend a product, I shall make it clear.

I. Temporary Color

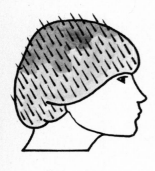

Color Rinses   (examples: Roux Fanci-full or Clairol's Picture Perfect Rinse). Can be an easy, quickie cover-up at home in between regular colorings but not by me in the salon. Easily accessible in your neighborhood drugstore, temporary rinses will brighten up your natural hair color, add a glow or intensify your own color. They are also an inexpensive and effective way of camouflaging gray hair. Most important, they will safely and easily shampoo out. These temporary products are just what the name implies; they are designed for you to use at home.

Don't expect drastic changes with a transparent temporary rinse. To cover gray in medium-brown hair, you must use a darker-brown rinse. Red tones will warm up brown shades but not create a new redhead. Blond rinses won't show up on dark hair because temporary rinses are transparent, and the natural color shines through.

RENN HINT: To cover gray, apply temporary rinse to freshly shampooed towel-dried hair with a cotton ball. Remember that the color usually looks darker before drying, blot with a paper towel before setting or blow drying.

Most temporary rinses are ready-mixed, but metallic-based rinses have to be mixed with water. *Beware*—the metallic salts can oxidize and change color, especially over previous color treatments or permanent waves. Highlights or streaked hair can turn out a disastrous green. Darker shades tend to rub off on your pillow.

There is a disadvantage to temporary rinses. These rinses coat the hair. Although they do wash out, they sometimes kill the shine and too much rinse will make the hair heavy and gummy. To get your $2.50 worth, know what temporary rinses can and can't do.

Color Sticks or Crayons   (example: Roux Color Crayons). Found in beauty-supply houses and some drugstores. As easy to apply as a crayon to a coloring book, color sticks fall into the temporary-color category and should be used only between color touch-ups. Apply on damp hair where new growth is beginning to show. This is *not* an all-over color. It is a quick touch-up or camouflage for home use only. It shampoos out. Color choice is limited. Pick the shade nearest your own hair. Light brown can be used for all light-brown to blond shades.

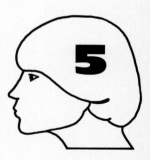

RENN HINT: Apply a small amount of crayon to new growth and blend with your fingertip. For darker shades, of course, you'll need to apply more.

2. Semi-Permanent Color

(No-peroxide color that coats the hair and covers gray, but which will fade with each shampoo and does *not* lighten your natural color)

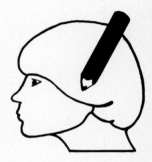

Five-Week Rinse Type   (examples: Clairol's Loving Care, Clairol's Happiness). Strictly designed for home use, with easy application (like applying shampoo), this product contains no peroxide but can "wash" away gray or warm up dull, lifeless hair. Most of these rinses contain built-in conditioners to protect the hair while processing.

The five-week rinses don't penetrate the hair shaft, but slightly coat it, so the hair takes on more body and texture. I find warm-brown shades are the most successful. Ash shades tend to build up after several applications and may become drab and dull.

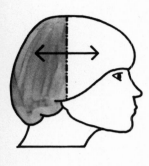

Single-Process (examples: Revlon's Young Hair NCT and Clairol's Beautiful Browns). This is the newest and most sophisticated of the *no-peroxide* five-week rinse. I use this type of color the most in the salon as a replacement for the tints with peroxide and I recommend them to you at home. Unlike other five-week rinses, the new semi-permanent color not only coats the hair shaft but has a 5 percent penetration to give more lasting results. It also comes in a wider range of colors than the other five-week rinse products. For these reasons I find these products give me the best results for my clients in the salon. With a single application this product will cover gray, will make your natural shade of hair richer, or will darken tones that are faded from too much sun. All this is done without peroxide and without the worry of oxidation that makes color turn brassy. I feel that since you have a choice you should use color that is better for your hair and that needs less maintenance. This is it!

With this product you get a small bottle of color with a packet of crystals, which you mix together by gently shaking them in a plastic applicator bottle. With one hand, squeeze the color out of the bottle onto your head, massaging the color gently into the scalp and hair with the thumb of your other hand.

> **RENN HINT: No-peroxide products tend to be thinner than those with peroxide, and care should be taken during application. Use just enough of the product to cover the hair but not so much that it runs down your face. A small paintbrush or tint brush can be used to go back over the color at the hairline to guard against drips.**

Apply the color just to the most resistant hairs—usually the gray or the new growth closest to the scalp. Allow color to process for 25 minutes before working through the rest of the hair for an additional 10 to 15 minutes. Timing will vary from product to product, so every five minutes wipe off the end of a strand of hair with a wet towel to determine desired depth of color. Remember, dry or permed, hair will grab the color much

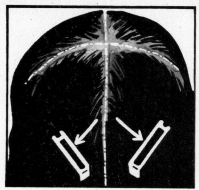

Section hair in 4 parts from center of crown; use clips if needed.

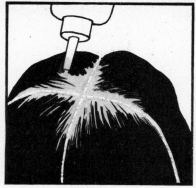

Outline the four partings with color mixture from applicator; then apply to each section of scalp.

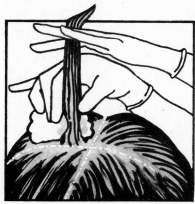

After application apply color to full strand, and test to determine color depth and coverage. Note: wear protective gloves!

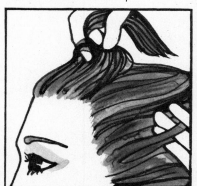

Work color through rest of hair for the last few minutes.

more quickly and always looks darker when it's wet. Always be sure to read all package instructions concerning that product's application and timing.

> **RENN HINT: Single-process color can create sophisticated and professional highlighting effects if your natural color is turning gray. The overall color tends to take lighter on those gray hairs and darker on your dark hairs.**

NOTE: This product cannot lighten; only peroxide products can do that. This is why I like to add natural-looking highlights for a lighter look rather than color the entire head. If you're growing gray you'll have natural highlights. If your hair is one color, I'll show you later how to add highlights.

Most color products carry a cautionary instruction about the possibility of an allergic or sensitive reaction to the product. You should do a patch test at least 24 hours before the application of color. Follow package instructions.

I have found that some people who are allergic to peroxide tints are not allergic to some of the five-week rinses. If you are one of those who are allergic to peroxide colors, you may be one of the lucky ones!

3. Permanent Color

Color Tint   (examples: Miss Clairol Color Bath, L'Oréal's Preference). This single-process hair coloring is also known as penetrating tint or simply hair dye. It is called permanent color because the structure of the hair is changed when the product penetrates into the cortex layer of the hair shaft, but it does fade with time. Color-tint colors can lighten hair, darken hair and cover gray.

Basically, this technique involves applying a mixture of the product with an equal amount of 20-volume peroxide, either liquid or cream. See illustration. This product is applied in the same way as the single-process semi-permanent color. Processing time varies from product to product.

RENN HINT: Single-process tint should be used only when your natural color is objectionable to you (for instance, too gray). The change in structure means hair feels thicker, but single-process tints must be renewed every four or five weeks because of new growth at the roots and fading or brassiness at the ends. The more drastic the change, the more trapped you are with maintenance and the added risk of overprocessed hair. You either apply new color—first to the new growth and then working through to the faded ends in the last few minutes of processing—or face a lengthy and ugly growing-out process.

RENN HINT: To prevent staining of the skin around your hairline, which occasionally happens (particularly with the darker shades), massage a small amount of cold cream right up to the hairline, being very careful not to cover any small hairs that you intend to color. If, however, any stains do occur, you can easily remove them by mixing a small amount of color with your shampoo and gently rubbing the mixture into the hairline, with a cotton ball *before shampooing* the entire head.

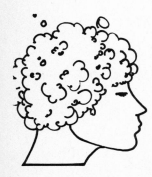

Shampoo-In Permanent Color   (examples: Clairol's Nice 'n Easy, Revlon's Colorsilk). Also a penetrating tint, this is different from single-process (or hair tint) color because the application (simplified for home use) is worked through the entire hair like a shampoo, left on for only 20 minutes, and then rinsed out. The advantage is that for touch-ups you repeat the shampoo process instead of making tricky touch-ups as in single-process color.

> **RENN HINT:** The technique is simple, but the ends of the hair may become increasingly porous with each new all-over application and may tend to grab color, making them too dark or too brassy.

Two-Process, or Blonding (also called Bleach and Toner and is not recommended). This process is synonymous with the Jean Harlow/Marilyn Monroe platinum-blond look. If this kind of blonde has more fun, she also pays for it in time, money and trouble. Those pastel shades of blond don't come easy. They are achieved through two time-consuming steps which can be damaging to hair and scalp and must be repeated regularly—bleaching and toning.

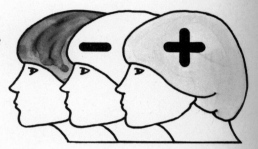

In the first step (or bleach-out), one part lightener or bleach (usually blue) is mixed with two parts of 20-volume liquid peroxide. The bleaching process usually takes 30 minutes to an hour.

In the second step, the toner is never applied until the hair is pale yellow in color and also porous enough to take the toner. The toner is mixed equally with 20-volume peroxide and applied to damp hair. After the correct pastel shade is achieved, the hair is rinsed and conditioned.

This is a definite two-part process. No one should be caught dead in the outlandish raw bleach-out color, but it's staggering how often women are allowed to walk out of a salon in this garish condition. And too many people attempting this process at home decide against the toner because the scalp has become overly sensitive to the bleach-out. But for the sensitive scalp, a new no-peroxide toner can be used instead.

> **RENN HINT:** No-peroxide toners can be used safely at home to tone down unwanted brassiness or turn on faded blondes. My favorite is Clairol's Born Blonde Toner (no-peroxide) Winsome Wheat. It is used like a shampoo, right out of the bottle with no mixing, because the crystals aren't necessary. I leave it on for 5 minutes to pick up blond tones and 10 minutes for darker brown shades.

Even in a salon under the best conditions, this two-process bleaching can be painful enough to bring tears to the client's eyes. Whether you are bleaching in a salon with professionals, or at home, repeated applications may cause severe breakage of hair. Permanent waves, electric rollers, curling irons and blowers sometimes spell instant disaster for overprocessed and weakened hair.

The return to the thirties and forties look in fashion may encourage women to reconsider the look of two-process hair coloring, but I haven't recommended or done a double-process in years. As a matter of fact, I salvage several of these a week. I feel that it chains a woman to expensive and time-consuming color, and that it does not fit into the lifestyle of today's woman. If you are already a two-process blonde and want to escape, try reverse streaks or highlights for a more natural-blond look.

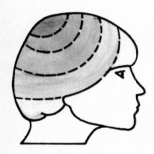

Metallic Compound Color Formula   (example: R.D. for Men, Grecian Formula—a definite *no-no*). This is used mainly by men, but hair is hair and the user will find the hair turning gradually darker with daily application of this clear liquid. It is applied right out of the bottle with a comb or brush like a hairdressing. No magic fountain of youth here. With daily use the color gradually gets darker and darker. Roots still grow in gray or white, but telltale new growth is hidden through repeated applications. With continued use, long hair tends to take on metallic highlights, and how natural the new color appears is a matter of opinion; I think the color looks obviously dyed. *Remember:* this is a permanent color, which I do *not* recommend.

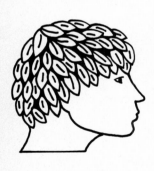

Henna   (permanent vegetable tint). There's nothing new about henna. Even Cleopatra is said to have used this vegetable tint, which made a resurgence in the 1960's when everyone was searching for "natural" products. It is natural, all right. This red-brown to orange-brown tint is made from the leaves of *Lawsonia inermis,* a shrub that grows in Asia and the Far East. Although henna is natural and organic, its results often look artificial. Most people would be put off if they only realized that henna is a permanent tint.

For starters, *never* use henna on hair already treated with a permanent hair color and *never* permanent wave over henna.

Henna has a tendency to build up on the hair, an added-body plus for fine hair, but disastrous for medium or curly hair, which begins to look unnaturally coarse and to feel unnaturally dry.

Henna is reputedly a temporary color, fading away gradually and leaving no growth line. But you might as well know the truth. It rarely does. I hate the obvious hennaed look and never use it in the salon.

Some Persian hennas have been so refined that the resulting shades are soft burgundies, but only the most experienced professional hairdresser can be sure that henna results will look as natural as the product promises. Too many hennas produce a harsh red glow, particularly garish over gray.

RENN HINT: But if henna you must, remember that the only healthy henna is the no-color or neutral henna, which gives body to fine hair and protects hair from the ravages of summer sun. Why else do you think Cleopatra used it on the Nile?

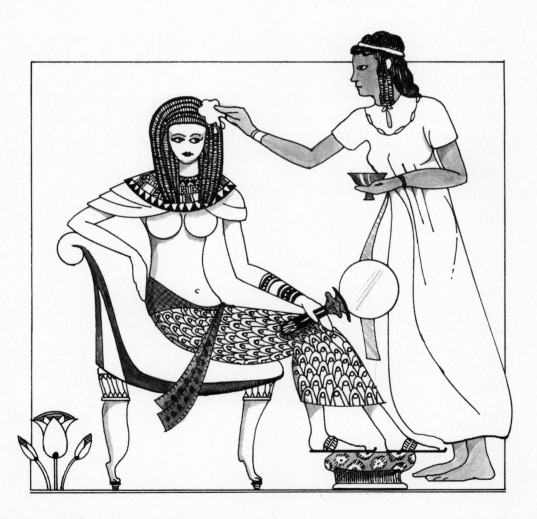

RENN'S
Natural Henna Conditioning Treatment

6 oz. powdered neutral henna (usually found in drugstores
      or health-food stores)
4 oz. plain yogurt
6 oz. hot pure water (not boiling)
1 egg yolk

Directions: In a large bowl, combine henna with hot water
to make a spreadable paste—add more water if needed.
Blend in the yogurt and egg yolk. Let mixture cool a little
so as not to burn your head, and apply evenly all over
your head like a treatment. At this time, a plastic Baggie is
placed over the head for about 25 minutes (without heat).
Rinse well and then shampoo.

Now hair will have new shine and added body, and this is
what henna is all about.

> **RENN HINT: This can be used every other month. It should not be
> used just before regular coloring treatments, but in between as a
> pick-me-up, for added body and shine.**

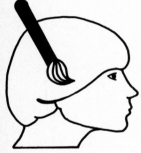

Hair Painting (example: Clairol's Quiet Touch). About
five years ago a kit was introduced that allowed you at home
to paint shiny glints of light or diffused highlights into your
natural (not dyed) hair color. Don't confuse hair painting with
frosting or streaking. Hair painting is far more subtle and should
only be done two or three times a year. I think, when done
correctly, hair painting is one of the quickest and simplest
methods to get shinier and more "sunlit" hair. With a
hair-painting kit I suggest painting tiny strands of hair, but only
touching the top layer of your hair. Work slightly away from
both the front line and your part for a natural effect.
    You can paint your hair successfully alone, but why not
make it a party with a friend? Kits are usually packaged for two
separate applications.

> **RENN HINT: Paint a few more lights around the face, less in back
> for a sunlit look. Darker hair tends to take on an artificial look if
> painting is made too light, so use care when painting. Redheads
> can use hair painting for golden highlights.**

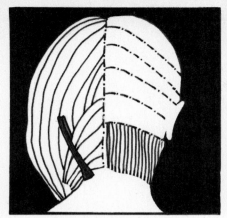

Section hair for application.

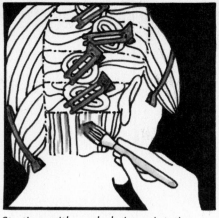

Starting with underhair, paint tiny strands to be lightened.

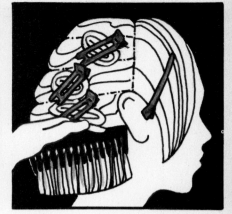

Gently comb through painted section and repeat process, working to crown.

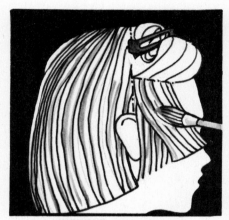

Need pointed paintbrush.

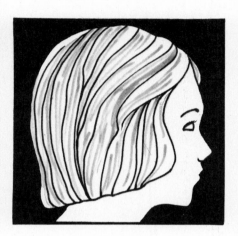

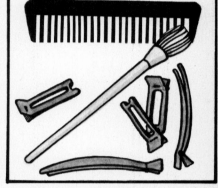

Supplies needed: comb, paintbrush, clips.

To retouch hair painting, after four or five months, simply fill in slightly as the hair grows out. Take care not to brush lightener over hair previously treated. Pomade or hair cream can protect previously painted strands.

Underplay when in doubt. (Test a strand of underneath hair for a quick look at what the results will be.) You can always do more later when surer of both the effect you want and of your application skills.

Frosting   Started by Marcel in Paris in the fifties, frosting quickly spread to the home circuit. The French wrapped individual strands of hair in foil. Americans simplified the procedure and cut the processing time in half just by developing a frosting cap and subsequently introducing home products.

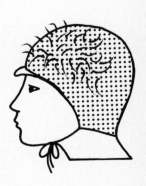

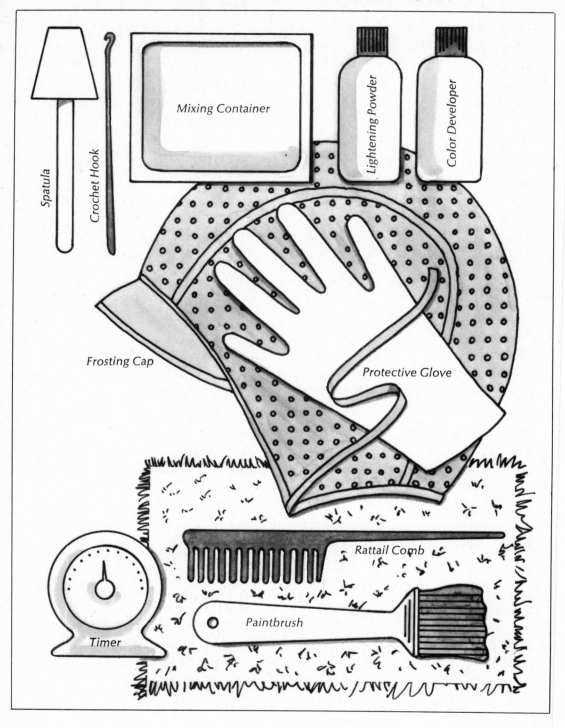

The frosting cap has been constantly improved. The early shower-caplike bonnets (still on the market) were followed by two-layer contour swim caps that have eliminated the danger of "bleeding" of bleach onto untreated hair inside the cap. Tiny strands of hair are pulled through the cap with a crochet hook and a lightener mixed with 20-volume peroxide is applied. The best caps are transparent, allowing you to see where a part or hairline will be as you pull out strands of hair for processing.

Frosting appears to lighten all the hair, but actually not all the hair is processed. Unfortunately, the look that has become synonymous with frosted hair is completely overdone and appears similar to that of the unnatural two-process procedure.

You can easily frost your hair at home, but there is always the danger of capturing that old-fashioned look of an almost all-over blond or blond shade highly contrasting with your dark hair. Or instead of looking blond, you may look gray. And a week or two later when your natural color screams out at the roots—you'll find yourself as trapped in color processing as the peroxide blonde.

But you can frost your hair the right way—and easily—at home. It is among the most versatile of methods if you know how to adapt the process to your individual needs—in other words, how to make it work for you.

New Highlighting Technique by Customizing Your Home Frosting Kit   (examples: Clairol's Frost & Tip, Revlon's Frost & Glow, L'Oréal's Frosting Kit). Change old-fashioned frosted hair into modern highlighting techniques. Farewell, frosting—hello, highlighting! If your kit comes with a plastic crochet hook, replace it with a metal one. (Plastic hooks are likely to break in mid-process.) Metal hooks are not only durable, they speed up the chore of pulling hair through the cap. They can be purchased in various sizes. The smaller the hook, the more delicate the effect. I recommend a No. 7 or 8 for the most subtle, desirable and complimentary effects. Use the plastic spatula *only* to mix the powder and liquid.

Do not apply the mixture to your hair with the spatula. Use a one-inch paintbrush, which you can buy at any hardware or dime store. The spatula only mats the hair, preventing an even distribution of the lightener and forcing the bleach and bleach fumes through the frosting holes to the scalp. You don't want to pack the hair—particularly long hair—down to the cap.

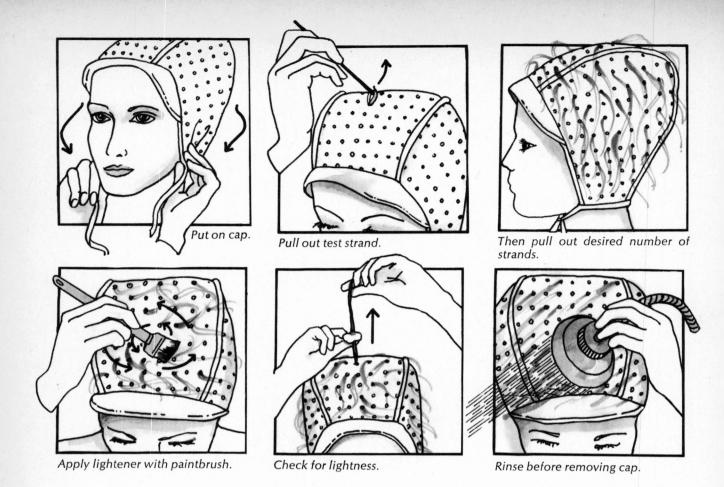

Put on cap.

Pull out test strand.

Then pull out desired number of strands.

Apply lightener with paintbrush.

Check for lightness.

Rinse before removing cap.

RENN HINT: For evenness of color, gently lift hair slightly away from the cap with a rattail comb to allow air to circulate through the hair. Use no heat, hair dryer, blower (or especially the plastic covering included in the kit) to speed up the process. Extra heat only forces the process out of control.

Customizing your equipment is not the only way you can tailor a standard frosting kit to meet your color needs. *Timing* is the key to the correct shades. Contrary to kit instructions, blondes wanting to go even blonder with gold-beige highlights should leave the lightener on only 10 minutes. Medium-brown hair needs about 20 minutes to achieve dark-blond highlights; dark brown needs only 15 minutes for red-brown, gold or toast shades. If you have dark-brown hair, forget about platinum shades. The effect is aging, unflattering and hard to maintain. Redheads should use the lightener for only 10 minutes for red-gold glints.

Even less time is required for more subtle brightening, and with proper timing you can achieve the correct shade in one simple process, eliminating the need for a toner, which tends to fade off anyway. Timing is the key to success. By cutting the time short, you won't have that obvious frosted look. What you will have is a softer, more subtle effect that only improves as it is growing out. Advantages of this new, natural, understated look are:

1. The sun brings out even more highlights rather than turning the new color brassy.
2. You have almost no growth lines to cope with, as you do with more extreme coloring processes.
3. You can forget worries about overlapping the color from touch-up to touch-up.
4. You will spend far less time processing your hair and dramatically cut down the chances of damaging it through overprocessing.
5. You will play up your skin tones as well as your natural hair color.

Always test a sample before beginning. You may think testing is a bore and a waste of time, but remember—testing is how professionals achieve the right results and eliminate the guesswork.

For the test, put on the frosting cap and pull out only a strand or two of hair in the crown. Mix a small amount of lightener and apply to the strands. Brunettes wanting simply a natural glow to brighten dull one-dimensional hair will usually achieve exactly that result in only 5 minutes. Medium-brown heads wanting brown on brown or lighter gold highlights need only 10 minutes of processing. And redheads generally need 5 minutes for a brighter red tone, 10 minutes for red-gold highlights. Dark blondes usually require 15 to 20 minutes to get that summer look, no matter what the weather is outside.

After the processing time, wipe the lightener off with a wet towel and towel-dry. Do not remove the cap yet. At this point, take a careful look to decide if you've allowed the proper amount of processing time. Dark brown should be shaded to a lighter red brown, brown to gold, blond to gold or ash. If additional lightness is desired, or if too much red is apparent, reapply bleach for five minutes and check. After rinsing and towel-drying, remove the cap and comb the test strands back into the rest of the hair. If testing achieved the predicted results, proceed with the rest of the hair. If not, proceed, but

HIGHLIGHT TIME CHART

	START →	TIME →	FINISH
	BRUNETTES — WANTING NATURAL GLOW, SUBTLE RESULTS.	5 MINUTES	BRIGHTENS ONE-DIMENSIONAL DULL HAIR.
	REDHEADS	5 MINUTES	BRIGHTER RED TONE/SUBTLE
	BLONDES	10 MINUTES	GO BLONDER WITH GOLD-BEIGE HIGHLIGHTS
	MEDIUM BROWNS	10 MINUTES	BROWN-ON-BROWN HIGHLIGHTS LIGHTER GOLD
	REDHEADS	10 MINUTES	RED-GOLD HIGHLIGHTS
	DARK BLONDES	15–20 MINUTES	SUMMER-LOOK
	MEDIUM BROWNS	20 MINUTES	DARK-BLOND HIGHLIGHTS
	DARK BROWNS	15 MINUTES	RED-BROWN, GOLD OR TOAST SHADES
	DARK BROWNS	FORGET IT!	PLATINUM

with the knowledge that you will leave the lightener on for a shorter time if test results were too severe, longer if the color wasn't achieved.

> **RENN HINT:** Remember that the new color of this individual strand might seem a bit too intense (or red) but keep in mind that when the strands blend with the rest of your darker hair, the new tone will blend and complement the old color, since only 25 to 30 percent of your total head of hair has been colored.

Before putting the cap back on, brush your hair straight back unless you normally wear a part, in which case, comb into your usual style. Hair coloring should complement the hair style, so decide on your hair style *before* coloring. Many dollars have been left on the cutting-room floor. Now, pull hair through the cap, always taking care to be a fraction away from the part and from the hairline. This technique helps to soften your natural color as it grows out. Pull out only a minimum of hair strands through each hole to keep the overall effect underplayed and natural.

Apply bleach sparingly, beginning at the crown and working in a circular fashion around the head until you cover all exposed hair. When too much lightener is applied, the chance of color leaking (or bleeding) through the cap increases. Besides, you only have to coat the hair slightly to achieve the desired effect. Too much lightener will create "hot spots"!

RENN HINT: For color framing when you want only highlights around your face, pull hair through the cap around only the front part of the head to about three inches back from the hairline, and apply the kit lightener. Timing corresponds to the lightness required for your skin tone. A glowing halo effect that is missing in an all-over lightening would then be the result.

These suggestions are made for the women whose hair has not begun to gray. But heads getting their own "natural" frosting may find that the standard frosting process of even my variations no longer work for them. The effect is muddy instead of glowing because gray hair can't take on blond tones. To brighten your light-gray shade, pull your hair through the frosting cap and apply a single-process or permanent color instead of the frosting lightener. Pick a gold-blond shade (Clairol's Golden Apricot) and leave it on for 30 minutes. As in the standard frosting process, rinse off color before removing cap.

If you have darker shades of gray hair, or if your hair is salt and pepper, play up your natural gray by streaking with a

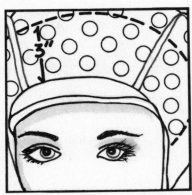

Pull out strands in front only.

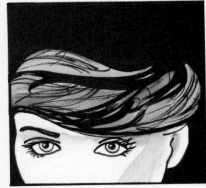

Result: glow around face.

brown single-process color to match your natural dark color. Pull hair through frosting cap and apply a dark-brown color, following the directions on the package for timing.

About 50 percent of your old gray hair will be eliminated as you add new sparkle and dimension.

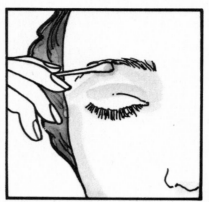

Keep eye closed during application.

Coloring Eyebrows and Eyelashes

Eyebrows are very important to facial expressions as well as for framing the eyes. They should be slightly lighter than your all-over hair color, in order to play up your eyes. Brows that are too dark and coarse can be made softer just by a slight lightening, and you won't have to tweeze constantly. I do not like the no-brow look that comes from bleaching them too much; it gives one a vacant, staring look.

Remember dark brows bleached too light can turn orangy. For lightening eyebrows I use one-part Clairol's Ultra-Blue lightener with two-parts 20-volume peroxide. Apply with a small brush or Q-tip. Leave it on a few minutes and then wipe off and check the color. If the desired look is not light enough, apply again for another short time. The idea is to lighten only slightly, not to change drastically. This procedure has to be done every few weeks, but is surely easy enough to keep up at home. Don't use harsh facial bleach such as Jolene bleach, as it works too quickly and usually turns too blond or orangy. If your brows are naturally too light, turning gray or just an undesirable shade, you might have to use a color, not a lightener. For this, a special color just for lashes and brows should be used, such as Roux's Lash-N-Brow tint. This is a vegetable tint and not a dye, made especially for brows and lashes. In most cases, only the brown color should be used, for just a few minutes so that they don't get too dark. Never use black for brows. Follow package instructions. *Never* use the same color product that you use on your hair for *brows.* It can be damaging if you get it in your eyes.

For lashes, black tint can be used, but I suggest that this specialized service be done only by a professional. Even I couldn't dye my own eyelashes.

In all these techniques you want what works for you. You want to give the hair body, texture, tonal qualities, shine, a play of light and a natural look that is always in style. This is the look that I try to achieve day after day in the salon—beautiful, healthy, natural-looking hair is timeless.

With a little time, a little education and not much money, you can create, at home, color tailor-made for you. But you will find that color after calculation, not by chance.

To simplify purchasing for you, here are the products that I use and that I recommend for you. Notice that Columns 1, 2 and 3 are different brands but equivalent.

Single-Process Five-Week Rinse No-Peroxide Colors

Revlon's Young Hair NCT	Clairol's Beautiful Browns	Clairol's Happiness Foam In Hair Color
Blonde 20	None	None
Light Brown 48	Light Ash Brown B08D	Light Warm Brown 910
Medium Brown 49	Medium Golden Brown B11W	Golden Brown 916
Auburn 30	Light Reddish Brown B09W	None

Highlighting

Clairol's Frost & Tip Highlighting Kit
L'Oréal's Conditioning Frosting Kit
Revlon's Frost & Glow

Hair painting

Clairol's Quiet Touch Hair-Painting Kit
L'Oréal's Brush-On Highlighting Kit

Corrective Hair Color – Fixing It

Dozens of people come to me each week with tales of woe, asking me about damaged hair and how to correct it. Why did it turn green from a chlorine pool? How can I stop my hair from breaking? How can I get out of this rut of having to do my roots every three weeks? What can I do?

Remember: it takes a lot of time and a lot of damage to ruin your hair. You can make it look 100 percent better in a short time by correcting the color, but it might take months to restore the condition, even with treatments and very gentle care. If you insist on being a long-hair person, it could take over a year for the old color and old damage to grow out.

The following are the most frequent questions my customers ask me in my salon. I expect they will be questions you might ask me too.

I use a one-process shampoo-in permanent color. How can I keep it from turning red?

Permanent dyes contain peroxide, which changes color from the effects of the sun and from oxidation. Use a semi-permanent color that has no peroxide, will cover gray and will last as long as so-called permanent tints. Always use one shade lighter than your natural color; this keeps the color looking natural, especially if you are trying to cover gray. Stay away from ash shades in no-peroxide tints, as they tend to build up on the hair and might acquire an unnatural, smoky-green cast. Warm browns, auburns, and honey blonds work best.

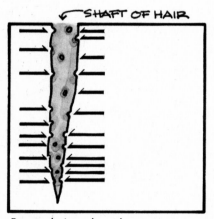

Porous hair grabs color.

RENN HINT: The ends of your hair are usually more porous, so keep the color off the ends until the last few minutes of processing time. Take a test strand and apply the color on a full lock of hair—from scalp through the end. After ten minutes wipe color off with a wet towel, and check to see if the ends are dark enough. Adjust processing time accordingly.

I don't color my hair at all; it is naturally blond, but it gets a greenish cast after too much dunking in a chlorine pool. Do I have to start dyeing my hair or just stay out of the water?

The following tip is for anyone whose hair turns a strange color from pool chemicals, whether the hair is natural, tinted, frosted or bleached. Use the old no-peroxide hair-color trick again, but this time a pale-blond color (Revlon's Young Hair

NCT #20 Blonde) is used all over the hair for about ten minutes. Not long enough to change the color but just long enough to take out the green cast. If stronger medicine is needed—especially if your hair is damaged or permed—use a hot-oil treatment that will lift some of the stain. Follow the oil treatment with the no-peroxide color mentioned above. The color can't hurt your hair, as it has no peroxide. Usually the darker the hair, the longer the blond color has to stay on to remedy the problem.

My henna is growing out; it has faded, but now my few gray hairs are orange. Help!!

Never use a permanent dye or peroxide tint over henna. The semi-permanent, no-peroxide color again comes to the rescue. Since semi-permanent color coats the hair, as henna does, the faded ends can be matched to your natural color by choosing the color most like the natural shade. Drugstores or beauty-supply houses have color charts to help you decide on the correct shade.

> **RENN HINT:** If your hair is gray, use a color product that is one shade lighter, so that the gray hairs after coloring are not as dark as your natural color but will look like highlights instead of dyed hair. This method will also work over dark or black henna, which usually gets a greenish cast when it starts to fade. Auburn or reddish-brown shades work best.

I frosted my hair and that is exactly what it looks like, old and gray. What can I do to fix it without further damaging my hair?

If your natural hair is dark brown and you have white frosting in it, of course it will make you look old. This look is a mistake even on light-colored hair. The damage is done, now let's fix it with semi-permanent products. If your natural hair color is medium to dark brown, use a warm-brown semi-permanent color over the frosting, which will give you natural-looking highlights while it takes away the gray. For lighter-brown shades use a honey or golden-blond no-peroxide toner (Clairol's Born Blonde Happy Honey) to cover over the frosted look. If you have red or auburn-colored hair, use a toast-blond toner to help out.

RENN HINT: Frosted hair is usually porous and is sometimes damaged, meaning that it will take color more quickly. After reading package instructions, apply color all over the head, without fear (no-peroxide, remember). Check after half of the prescribed processing time. Since the toner is formulated to take only on prebleached hair, it will only color the frosted part, so don't worry about its changing your natural color. It can also pep up old frostings between treatments or while it's growing out.

I have been bleaching my hair for years and it never turns out the same color twice. To make matters worse, it is breaking and looks like straw. How can I get out of this constant maintenance and still have a blond look?

If your natural color growing in is light brown or dark blond, the solution is simple.

You might use a darker tone of blond or go into highlighting. But if your roots are dark brown or look black to you, more work is needed to put your hair on the road to recovery. First of all, the thought of changing very light hair to a darker shade is enough to set a lot of people off, right there. But I think it's something you're going to have to live with.

If you are really a brunette, a *reverse-streaking* process (putting darker contrasting streaks throughout solid blond hair) is the only way to get you out of this endless bleaching, still giving you a blond look, while your healthy new hair is growing in. In a few months you should be able to start highlighting the new growth. For the reverse-streaking process, I honestly recommend that you call on a good colorist, one that is also patient and sympathetic. He should use a no-peroxide color, a shade darker than the natural color of your hair growing in (two-thirds dark color mixed with one-third auburn color to keep the brown from going ash and looking drab). Starting underneath and working toward the front, your colorist should pick up small strands, apply the brown mixture and wrap the strands in aluminum foil to keep the color from running or dripping onto the rest of the damaged, blond hair. The best time for this process is about three weeks after your last bleach touch-up. If your hair has grown out too far, you might get one last bleach touch-up and get ready for your new change three weeks later. The final look should be an overall darker-blond color because of the darker contrasting streaks. This will make it look much more natural. Best of all, the roots won't be apparent for weeks and weeks. Wait as long as possible, meanwhile giving your hair lots of conditioning, and then add lighter highlights to the *new* growth. You can do this three or four times a year instead of every three weeks as before, so you will end up not only with new *hair* but also with a new liberated *you.*

> **RENN HINT:** Don't let anyone talk you into dyeing all of your bleached hair dark brown first and then streaking or adding blond highlights over that, as the permanent dye will oxidize and fade in a few weeks, and you'll be right back where you started. Also, bleaching over hair that is already damaged only harms the hair. I have seen successful reverse streakings done at home with a frosting cap, but if your problem is as severe as some I've seen, let a pro get you back on the road to recovery first, then choose your new look and proceed at home.

I have been streaking my hair successfully, but recently the color seems to keep getting lighter and lighter, and now I even have ugly roots as it is growing in. What should I do?

When streaks get too light or too many streaks are taking away contrast needed to look natural, I either add contrast by putting in a few darker streaks (as in reverse streaking) or by using a darker-blond no-peroxide color on the entire head, knowing that it will only take on the prelightened streaks, toning them down in-between color treatments. Then add fewer highlights or streaks when your hair needs coloring later. This way your hair looks better while it is growing out and it will be healthier as well when new highlights are needed.

> **RENN HINT:** Not all of your hair has to be highlighted every three months. I often do a full head only once or twice a year and do small amounts or fill-ins in between. This keeps the color fresh-looking and your hair in perfect condition, without worrying about sun or fading color.

I use a permanent color on my hair to make it a brighter red. At first the color is fine, but it begins to fade quickly and get very brassy. My friends call me a "tacky redhead" . . . How can I get a softer color that won't fade so quickly?

Your color formula had too much lightener or bleach in it and not enough color or red tone (such as a shampoo-in tint). Start by considering the fact that your hair has become overporous because of excessive coloring and, as a result, has difficulty holding color. Try using a darker tone for a while, and don't put the mixture on the damaged ends until the color has taken on the new growth. Most permanent tints color and lighten at the same time, which means that touch-ups should be done *first* on the new growth *only.* After 20 minutes the color can be worked through the rest of the hair, and then checked after 10 minutes. If the color isn't dark enough, leave it on and keep checking every few minutes, until it's ready.

> **RENN HINT:** For the first 20 minutes of application the color strength of the solution is strongest, and will lighten the most. After the color has been on your scalp for this amount of time, it is still strong enough to color your porous ends but not so strong as to damage them. A better, longer-lasting solution would be to use a no-peroxide semi-permanent color, like Revlon's Young Hair NCT Auburn 30. This would brighten natural tones but will not lighten them.

I have black hair and have been coloring it since I began to see a few gray hairs. It looks so unnatural and severe. Is there something else I can do instead of continuing this process?

The trouble with coloring hair black is that the dye makes the hair one flat color without any subtle highlights or shading, and this is what makes it look so artificial and hard. As we get older our skin tones fade and one should use a hair color a shade or two lighter. I would never, no, *never,* use black dye on anyone.

If you want a change, several things can be done. The easiest solution for you, and certainly the easiest on your hair, is to use a dark-brown color, preferably the no-peroxide kind, on your new growth *only,* leaving the ends alone, which should fade naturally. This way the color will gradually become lighter as it grows out, and there will be no quick change that would be difficult for you to get used to.

Do not bleach out all the old black dye and start from scratch. This drastic measure is not only costly but also very damaging to your hair. In fact, you might not have any hair left to recolor.

There *is* a dye-removal process, but it should be done by a color expert. A special dye-solvent color-remover product is mixed with peroxide and left on until the black dye has lifted several shades lighter. Next, the hair is shampooed and dried, and the new lighter hair—usually a hideous red or orange color after this process—is colored with a medium- or light-brown tint. With this process the dyed hair is not damaged nearly as much as with bleaching, and it also can be colored the new shade the same day.

RENN HINT: After the dye-removal process, hair is more porous and takes new color quickly and usually is a shade darker than desired. Use a lighter brown the first time, to be sure, and no-peroxide colors to retain the health of hair.

My hair is colored a medium-brown shade, and now that I am doing my touch-ups at home, the last three inches of my hair keep getting darker and darker. I even used a lighter shade than usual, but it is still dark. What will lighten the ends up enough to match the rest of my color?

Ends of hair grab the color after being overprocessed, and as a result they become porous. With a shampoo-in tint, you apply the color all over your head at each touch-up. What you should be doing is first apply the color to the new growth only, let that process, and then work the tint through the ends, gently coloring them for the last few minutes only. After the damage has been done, it is hard to lift tint from the darker ends. At first apply a hot-oil conditioner for about 20 minutes just to the ends. Most of the time the oil will lift a little color, and you will be getting a treatment at the same time. If the ends are still too dark, the oil treatment can be reapplied as many times as needed. If this doesn't work, highlight the ends only. This is done with the frosting-cap method. Pull the tiny strands through the cap and just brush the dark ends with the lightening mixture. Process for only a few minutes (checking them often) to lift them into a light brown or dark gold. This will give your one-process color extra zip as well, by giving your usual brown color more lights and more dimension.

RENN HINT: When you do your next color touch-up in a month or so, just the new growth needs coloring. If you have trouble applying the color to the back, ask a friend to help!

If your color has gotten brassy or too light from the sun, which usually doesn't happen with no-peroxide colors, the overall color can be toned down by mixing the remaining color (left over from your retouch application) with an equal amount of shampoo and by working this mixture through the rest of the hair. Check those porous ends often and don't let them get too dark. Sometime less than 5 minutes is all that is needed to freshen up a look.

Taking Care of Your Hair

The condition of your hair is everything. Just as our bodies need proper diet, vitamins and exercise to keep it going, hair needs a special regime to keep it going as well. Someone in poor physical condition will never have beautiful hair.

Color-treated hair is special and you should treat it as such, with frequent, gentle cleaning and regular conditioning. These conditioners need not be expensive, but they must be correctly prescribed products with ingredients that really do something to help your hair. There are many products that promise miracles but that do nothing to improve the condition. They just leave it smelling good. They can be good in a pinch, though, and we'll talk about them later.

Then there are the facts. A few years ago all the shampoos and conditioners were said to contain egg; next came the lemon craze and finally the herbal binge. It's amazing nowadays how anything containing herbs will sell. Do all these things really help the products? Of course not.

Hair that is damaged will always benefit from conditioning. Overprocessing from bleaching dries out the hair and makes it impossible to style or even to comb out when it is wet. Frequent conditioning treatments and the use of the new, more gentle type of hair coloring will make this problem much easier to live with until the condition is corrected.

You should know about different conditioners and when to use them. This knowledge will enable you to pick the right one to cure your individual problem. Remember, your hair color is very important to the total look of your hair, and the condition of your hair is what makes really beautiful color possible.

Shampoos

Always use a mild shampoo that is marked, "special for color-treated hair." Most shampoos contain harsh detergents that can fade color as well as dry out your hair. Most natural products do not contain detergents and usually list their ingredients on the container. These products seem to work best for people who have to shampoo often to keep their hair looking fresh and clean. In most cases only one shampooing is necessary to clean the scalp and hair. If your product does not lather much, it might be because your water is hard. Certain minerals in the water make it impossible to get a good lather, and that can result in not getting the hair clean or in not getting all the soap out. You can install a special water-softening system if this is a real problem for you.

Baby shampoo is said to be mild, but it does contain detergent. Lots of people swear by it and it doesn't seem to strip the color.

The top-selling pH-balanced shampoos are really an advertising gimmick. pH, meaning potential hydrogen, is the measurement of the alkaline or acid content of a solution. The pH Scale is between number one and number fourteen, with number seven being neutral. Hair is usually between number four and five, making it naturally acidic. A product would have to be extremely high either in acid or in alkali to make an important difference in your hair. A low-pH shampoo or conditioner is said to be best and most gentle, but it lacks the ability to lather, and it gives you the feeling of not getting your hair clean.

Dandruff shampoos should be used only if you have a problem. They contain tar or sulfur and will dry and strip your hair color. Try these treatments the week before you color or alternate them with more gentle, color-treated shampoos until the dandruff is gone. It is natural for a few flakes to be seen on your shoulder or brush, since this is just the wearing away of old scalp tissue. If your problem is critical, see a doctor, but I have found that Selsun Blue is just about the best product—and it is sold over the counter—for colored hair. If your hair is dry, follow all treatments with a good natural conditioner. Apply it only to the hair and *never* to the recently dandruff-treated scalp.

Rinses

A dandruff rinse is a liquid poured over the hair after shampooing. This product is usually stronger than the shampoo and runs off the scalp, but it is absorbed by the hair. Since the scalp is the problem area for dandruff, I feel that this rinse is not nearly so successful as the dandruff shampoo. And it is much harder on your hair and its color.

A cream rinse is not a true conditioner at all. It is a mixture that contains oil mixed with water and scents, and it makes your hair smell nice. It is rinsed over the hair after shampooing to enable you to comb out tangles. In no way does it restore damaged hair or help the condition.

A lemon or vinegar rinse is used to remove soap scum or residue left from either improper rinsing of shampoo or from hard water. Lemon and vinegar rinses are acid, which puts them low on the pH Scale. They might leave your hair feeling clean and shiny, but they are very drying to colored hair. Don't put lemon juice on your hair and then sit in the sun. If you have baby-fine hair, it might lighten a bit, but on most other hair textures and on dark colors lemon brings out unfavorable red tones. You'll end up with dry, brittle and sunburned hair.

A Sylk rinse is easy to use and one of the most professional rinses. It really *does* something, without harming or drying colored hair. You can buy it in beauty-supply stores. Sylk is primarily a water softener and you can use it after shampooing to remove all the soap. It will leave your hair more manageable, and, unlike most cream rinses, it will not leave it limp. Mix a teaspoon of powdered Sylk with warm water and work it through the hair as a final rinse. Since color-treated hair is usually porous and has a tendency to hold soap or conditioners, it often appears dull and lifeless and it takes forever to dry. If you have been afraid to condition because you couldn't ever rinse the conditioner out, your problem is solved—hair sparkles after a Sylk rinse. Professionals have been using Sylk for years, especially when clean hair is very important, such as before giving permanent waves or any other processes requiring clean hair.

Conditioners

Instant Conditioners are truly only a cosmetic for the hair. They may alter or temporarily change the texture of your hair, but they will wash right out and will not correct any problem you may have. Usually of a cream base, the instant conditioner contains ingredients that coat the hair shaft and replace lost oils with balsam, herbs or protein. Some come with lemon flavors, herbs, protein or even pH-balanced formulas, but that's simply to jazz them up for the big sell. The hair will comb more easily after this treatment and will feel much better, but no actual rebuilding of hair will occur. If the hair is overbleached or damaged, an instant conditioner—especially the balsam kind—is almost impossible to rinse out. However, if you use a very small amount, you can comb your hair easily and you will not run the risk of filling the porous hair with too much cream. If your hair is limp and dull after such a conditioning, or if you just can't get it out of your hair, try Sylk in the final rinse water. Follow it with a cold-water rinse to close the outside cuticle layer of the hair strand. This will make it easier to handle after the treatment.

If you are blessed with coarse hair or curly hair that needs to be softened or made more silky, then this can be a good conditioner for you. It makes the hair more limp, softer and more manageable for styling. Remember, this is only a temporary change, as your hair will soon revert to its original texture.

Penetrating Conditioners can be divided into two basic types: oil treatments and natural-ingredient conditioners with a cream base.

Oil treatments usually have a protein and mineral oil base and are highly refined so that they can be easily absorbed into the hair. The penetrating oil goes into the hair shaft and replaces the precious oils and nutrients that have been lost by overcoloring, sun damage or other problems. This is the best treatment for tinted (but not bleached!) hair which is of medium or coarse texture and which needs extra oil for repairing severe dryness. After you apply the conditioner—2 or 3 ounces only—you should, if possible, use a heat cap. First cover the hair with a plastic bag, then put the cap on loosely for about 20 minutes. The hair usually cannot absorb any more oil even if it is left on longer, and it tends to get gummy and hard to rinse. Never use more than medium heat. You should do this once a week for about six weeks. This oil treatment can lift and fade your color, but if you want your hair to be in better condition, the wait will be worth it.

A penetrating oil conditioner is not recommended if your hair is highly bleached and thus overporous and damaged. You will not be able to rinse it out, and it will leave the hair limp and oily. Also, I don't recommend a heat cap for bleached hair, as the weight of the cap combined with the heat could break fragile hair.

Oil treatments are very good for dry scalps too. If you have dry scalp, you can take a treatment every six weeks or so. It will make your hair shinier and will give it a healthy glow, and it will make your hair and your color easier to maintain.

Natural Conditioners are usually organic in composition and consist of a blend of such ingredients as bone marrow, vitamins, protein supplements and special minerals, all with a creamy base. Unrefined and totally natural, such conditioners don't even contain preservatives and some can be bought in health-food stores. Professionals, as well as actors and models, have been relying increasingly on organic properties for shampoos, conditioners and anything else useful for restoring hair. Natural conditioners penetrate into the hair shaft to replace lost moisture and therefore help return hair to its natural elasticity and health.

With this product it is not as important, as with the oil treatment, to use a heat cap.

> RENN HINT: You can use a hot wet towel, which gives extra-moist heat, just as a steamer machine does in expensive salons. The towel should be large enough to wrap around your head completely. It should not be so hot as to burn your scalp. As the towel cools, it can be replaced with another hot one, or you can heat up the same one again. You might feel that 20 minutes of this activity will send you out of your mind, but moist heat is really best for the hair. Caution: If you have highly bleached hair, do not use a very hot towel—instead use a warm treatment. Your hair will react very well. There is also something marvelous about the feel of the hot or warm towel around your head. You can use this time to clear your mind and to rebuild your hair.

Natural or organic conditioners come in liquid form and are packaged in small plastic or glass ampules; they contain, along with other ingredients, some type of placenta from lambs or other animals. There are several different formulas for damaged hair, and there is even one for extremely oily hair or dry hair. This type of conditioner is applied to the wet hair after shampooing, right out of the container, and is not rinsed out, unlike other conditioners. It is quickly absorbed into the hair and will not interfere with setting lotions or styling. It gives fine, limp hair more body and stops badly damaged hair from breaking. It is simple to apply. You can purchase it in shops or beauty-supply houses. Don't let its high price throw you; it is worth the money you pay. You do need a treatment after every shampoo until the damaged hair is restored to perfect health. A conditioner of this type does work.

> RENN HINT: If your hair is very short, use half a container and save the rest for the next time you wash your hair. I also recommend this conditioner for men. It is not messy to use and it gives protection for thinning hair. Several different companies make these conditioners, but the one that I see most in the drugstores is *Fermodyl,* which has different formulas for different problems. Ask for all the information where you purchase it and make sure that you are using the correct one for your problem.

Just about any hair-care problem can be helped with·these products that I've just described. A combination of conditioning treatments, a nondamaging method of hair coloring and the patience to allow the hair to grow will restore the look and feel you want. Remember: the color of your hair is only as good as the condition.

The Right Conditioner for You

Now that we know a little about the different types of conditioners and what they do, let's find out how to use them correctly in order to restore your problem hair and to give it new shine and vitality.

Normal hair is not dry or oily, but it does need a little help from time to time, just to keep it that way. Shampoo as often as needed with a mild, low-detergent, pH-balanced shampoo. If your hair is long and tangles after shampooing, use an instant conditioner to remove tangles and to give the hair body and texture. I like to follow all treatments with a final cold-water rinse to close the outside cuticle layer of the hair shaft and to give it more shine and luster. Use a very small amount of conditioner and if you find your hair dull and heavy, use a Sylk rinse after the conditioning.

If your hair is long or extra-long, you might find that just the ends get dry. If so, only apply the instant conditioner or deep-penetrating-cream natural conditioner to the dry part of your hair.

> **Renn Hint: Don't use a heat cap and don't pile your hair on top of your head if you are treating ends, as this will tend to get the normal hair oily. Confine the conditioning to just the part of the hair that needs the treatment. Normal hair will only need a special treatment each month or so, or after a permanent wave or straightening process, but don't worry, I have never known anyone who damaged her hair from too much conditioning.**

Oily hair needs less conditioning than normal hair in general, but blow dryers, hot rollers and overprocessing from perms or colorings can dry out even this hair. This can be a blessing, since oily hair can actually benefit from the drying properties and become more like normal hair. The ends might get a little drier, but if you condition from time to time after colorings and other processes, you can keep the dryness in check. Even henna, which I really don't trust, will sometimes leave oily hair with more shine, since it takes out some of the natural oils.

Dry hair is a problem, whether you color it or not, especially if it is fine in texture. For proper maintenance you should give it weekly treatments of a deep-penetrating, organic conditioner (René Furturer's Revitalizing Cream), using hot wet towels for about 15 or 20 minutes. *Do not use a heating cap,* as fine hair will tend to break from too much heat.

> **RENN HINT:** Alternate with treatment such as Fermodyl, which doesn't have to be rinsed out. This will give fine hair more body and shine, and will give more elasticity to dry, brittle hair.

By constantly conditioning fine hair and keeping it in shape, I have clients who are now coloring their hair who thought it would never be possible without doing a lot of damage. You can do the same.

Highly bleached hair that is breaking is, of course, the most difficult to restore. If that is your problem, you already know that it won't comb out after shampooing; it doesn't work with the new blow-dry styles, and that even rollers will leave ridges and marks on the hair after it is dry. Damaged hair takes much longer to dry because it has been made overporous, and the ends of the hair, like sponges, hold on to excess moisture.

You have to make several big decisions right now about the condition of your hair, while you are still lucky enough to have some. First, the color. Probably a double-process bleach and toner is what got you into this dilemma in the first place. You've already read how to have a blond look by reverse streaking, without the damage and time waste of bleaching, and you might as well start now. But your new look will only start to work for you as the condition of your hair improves. This won't happen overnight, but because your color has been improved with reverse streaks, you can go for a much longer time before you need color again. This will give you the freedom you need to grow new healthy hair, since you only need new highlights every few months instead of every three weeks. Now is the time to condition this damaged hair. Don't worry, your broken hair will grow back. You'd be surprised to know how many models have come to me with very damaged hair. They all have healthy hair now!

Shampoo only when you must, with a very mild shampoo without detergent, and made especially for bleached hair. Dilute it half with water to ensure proper rinsing. Do not use cream rinses or heavy cream-based instant conditioners, especially balsam. I do recommend Fermodyle, since it usually stops the breaking, is quickly absorbed into the hair shaft and doesn't need to be rinsed out. If the bleached hair is not quite so badly damaged, use a small amount of natural, organic conditioner with a hot towel—do *not* use a heat cap—for 10 minutes, followed by lots of rinsing with water turned on full force. A Sylk rinse wouldn't hurt to get the excess treatment out! And again, use a cold rinse. Blot with a thick towel and do not rub harshly, as this will only further damage or break the hair.

If your hair is hard to comb, just skip this step and don't comb it out until it is dry. Bleached hair loses its elasticity and may continue to break if you comb out tangles harshly. Hair is in its most delicate state wet, but dry hair can take more abuse. You can dry your hair with a medium-heat blower or under a cool dryer or just naturally by itself. When it is dry, free it from tangles by brushing gently with a natural-bristle brush or combing with a wide-tooth comb. Avoid anything *hot,* such as hot rollers, hot dryers or curling irons. The important thing now is to keep your old damaged hair in the best condition possible while the new hair grows in. This will allow the new look to take over the old. Trim away the dead ends frequently.

RENN HINT: **This is not the best time to start growing your hair long, as you should be cutting off the old hair as it is growing out. Keep the styling simple, and *no* perms or other processes for you until the healthy hair has grown in. It's a short time to wait for the reward of beautiful hair!**

Treatments That Go Hand in Hand With Coloring

Conditioners can actually help you to get the proper results from your color. If you are applying a single-process color and have a difficult time keeping the ends of the hair from getting too dark because of overporosity, apply a cream conditioner to the ends. This will protect them from getting dark. *Don't ever comb the color through.* Wearing protective gloves, gently work the color through the rest of the hair during the last 10 minutes of processing time. It might take a few minutes longer for the color to take on the ends, but keep checking by wiping off a strand with a wet towel until the color is developed.

RENN HINT: **If you find it difficult to get an even color because of past damage to your hair or because parts of your hair are lighter than others, apply the Fermodyle or René Furturer R.F. 13 treatment before you color, and dry it into the hair. Remember this**

treatment is not rinsed out; it will act as a filler to equalize the different porosities and will make the color take much more evenly. Process time may take a bit longer, but do a strand test to make sure.

If you have been using a semi-permanent color like Loving Care, you may be left with an ashy build-up or a greenish cast. Use a hot-oil treatment such as Clairol's Metalex, and apply to the discolored parts of your hair. Use a hot wet towel for 10 or 15 minutes. You might need a few of these treatments, especially if the problem is severe. There is no problem of added damage, since this is a very safe treatment. Remember to do this *before* the coloring.

>**RENN HINT: When you apply new color use a warmer tone and not an ash color, since it's the ash build-up you are trying to get rid of.**

The Metalex method will work on all hair colors from dark to white or gray hair. Nothing is uglier than white hair that gets a blue cast. The Metalex treatment will also help here, by lifting out the stain and giving it shine and good health. You can lift these stains or build-ups of color with a bleach mixture, but this is really an added chemical process, so I don't recommend it.

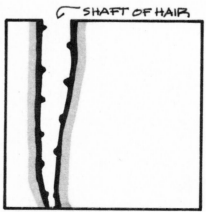

Fermodyl coating pores for even color.

Metalex can help out if your hair coloring doesn't seem to take, or doesn't cover the gray. This happens sometimes when hair is coated by color, or a build-up of hair sprays. Follow the directions on the Metalex bottle. You'll be surprised at how easily you'll get good results. Remember, there is always a reason why color doesn't take. Once you know how to correct it, and then do so, you'll find that your hair is easier to work on and that you'll get better results from the color. To say nothing of the health!

For Permanents   If your hair is colored and you can't get a successful permanent wave, before you try again start conditioning your hair way in advance. You'll end up with natural, softer hair instead of frizzy or overprocessed hair. Use R.F. 13 or a Fermodyle special lotion and carefully roll the hair around the perm rods, with the conditioner left in the hair to protect it from the chemical process. Use a special perm marked "for tinted or colored hair" and apply the wave lotion after the entire head has been wrapped in the perm rods.

> RENN HINT: The curl or wave should be three and one half times the size of the perm rods. The smaller the rods, the tighter the curls; the larger the rods, the less curl and the more body.

You can now perm highlighted or frosted hair successfully by protecting the streaks with a conditioner before the perm. Put the Fermodyle on wet hair, after you have shampooed gently, and then wrap the hair in permanent-wave rods. Use a color-treated perm lotion for the proper curl. Usually, if the normal hair is curled enough, the streaks will end up being overprocessed, and, conversely, if the lighter streaks have taken the curl properly, the normal hair will not be curled enough. Either way, uneven waves and tired curls are the result. If you first protect the streaks with the conditioner, all of your hair will take the perm evenly, just as one-textured hair would.

Beware of the "computer perms," which claim to give you the proper processing times. This gimmick will not work well if you have frosted hair or different degrees of porosity in your hair. A successful perm over colored hair is tricky, but it is certainly possible, if you know what makes it work.

For Hair-Painting Retouches   The first time you hair-paint it's really easy to get some nice little glints of light or subtle highlights with the painting kit, but you will find it isn't so easy to put in new lights without overprocessing the old ones. This can result in broken hair or streaks that are too light. Before you paint the new highlights (where the darker hair is growing in), paint the old lights with a thick cream conditioner, such as Clairol Condition, using the same little brush that comes with your painting kit. Wash the brush thoroughly and dry it on a towel. Now you are ready to paint in new lights, without the worry of overpainting, or of looking unnatural.

For Straightened Hair   If you feel that curly hair is your downfall and you simply cannot live with the natural curl that God gave you—the curl that other women with straight hair would die for—then and only then should you proceed with the straightening process. I have seen more broken and damaged hair resulting from straightening than from all other processes together. First of all, no matter what the condition of your hair, going perfectly straight will result in overprocessing. Curly hair can be relaxed, which will enable you to achieve a new look without destroying your hair. Colored hair is especially difficult to process, and a special gentle solution for fine or color-treated hair should be used. Be gentle with straightened hair, as it can break easily. You must replace its vitality with constant conditioning and gentle care.

> RENN HINT: After straightening, coloring can be difficult. The hair is now in a different state of porosity and will take the color much faster. If this process has faded the color, which sometimes happens, your color formula should be slightly lighter, as the new straightened hair will tend to "grab" and will get darker on the ends. Conditioner again can protect the ends from getting dark at the same time as it treats the hair.

Perms or straightening should be done *before* color, as they will fade or strip some color. The new color should not be done for a week or so, and should only be done after a good treatment. I could never say enough about conditioning treatments. They make my color work possible even on the most delicate and fragile hair. They just go hand in hand. Make them work for you too.

Special for Men

Why is it that when women see a few gray hairs they quickly cover them up for fear of appearing older, and when men turn gray, the same women say it looks distinguished? Well, that's beginning to end now. Men are discovering that hair color can work the same way for them—adding confidence, excitement and a youthful look! More men each year are coloring their hair. But men have to look natural at all times, even as the color is growing out. A man can't run the hundred-yard dash or give orders in his office with his roots showing. Why should he have to?

The market is now flooded with products marked "For Men Only." Cosmetics with fewer perfumes are designed to give him a suntanned look. There are complete lines of hair conditioners designed to improve looks and keep hair healthy at the same time. Hair-color products are now much more sophisticated, and many are especially designed with men's needs in mind. These are the ease-to-apply, no-peroxide shampoo-in formulas, which men can use in the privacy of their own bathrooms.

For years men have been coloring their hair for films and television and have been looking just great to us sitting at home. But hair that looks terrific on the screen usually looks reddish or brassy in real life, and the dark shades look very black and obviously dyed. Why does this happen? Too many color changes and too much peroxide are really the problems with actors' hair. Changing to no-peroxide tints will give a softer look to the color, as well as improve the condition of the hair. What's good for an actor should be good for any man!

Since men's hair is usually short, any color can look harsh if there are no highlights. Remember: even dark-brown hair has very subtle, light shadings.

Gray hair can be covered with a lighter-brown, no-peroxide tint, giving a highlighted look all in one process.

Hair that is getting darker with age can be brightened up with highlights that will grow out naturally, never look artificial and, above all, will not change color as other processes do.

In fact, with a little know-how and a lot of taste, men can use all the tricks and methods in this book, adopting them for their own use and needs. All care should be taken to always underplay each technique, and experimenting should be kept to a minimum. Study the chart and you will know exactly what will work for you, with the least amount of effort and virtually no experimentation.

How about Trying a Temporary Rinse to See How You'll Look?

If you have a few gray hairs that you would like to cover up, or if you would like to see what your very gray hair would look like if it were lighter brown or even blond, try on your new color just for fun. By using a temporary rinse, aware that it will completely wash out, you can get a notion of what a new color can do for your looks. Two of the best and most popular rinses on the market are Roux's Fanci-full and Clairol's Picture Perfect. The Roux Fanci-full rinses are easy to find in drugstores and have a good range of colors. The Clairol rinses can be bought in beauty-supply houses.

To cover a little gray if your natural hair color is dark to light brown, I suggest using Fanci-full color "Chocolate Kiss" right out of the container.

RENN HINT: Read the instructions first, but I believe it works best when applied with a ball of cotton. Hair is usually washed first, towel-dried and then the rinse is applied *just* to the gray hairs to be covered. Enough rinse should be used to coat the gray hairs, but too much will cause an unnatural feel to the hair and will only end up running down your face. After application, blot with an old towel or paper towel, comb into your usual style and let dry naturally or blow dry. Just like magic your gray hair is gone, you get to see what you look like *sans* gray hair and all for around two dollars!

If you have a lot of gray, or even a full head of gray hair, naturally the rinse should be applied to all of your hair.

RENN HINT: This takes a little more effort, but it must be done a little at a time by holding the bottle of rinse in one hand and massaging it into the hair with your other hand. Don't dump the entire bottle over your head. Lean over the bathroom sink during the first few applications. Soon you will be able to put the color on in the shower without looking.

Remember that this rinse is transparent and will dry lighter than it looks when it's wet, so don't get panicky when you see the wet color. Since rinses coat hair, they give new body to fine hair and will hold your hair in place without your having to use a lot of spray. A hard hair-spray finish is not very attractive; hair should move.

RENN HINT: The only hair spray on the market, as far as I'm concerned, is Clairol's Final Net. It is a liquid in a pump-applicator and should be used sparingly by spritzing in quick blasts, holding the container as far away as you can reach. Never apply so much that the hair becomes wet with the spray. It will end up looking like a wig.

If you don't want to cover your gray hair but have been wondering what you would look like as a blonde, try a blond rinse and see what happens. Roux's Fanci-full color "Gilded

Lilly,'' is just about the only rinse that has enough blond pigment to work on gray hair. Shake well and don't be surprised when it comes out of the bottle bright yellow; believe me, it won't look like that when it dries. Follow directions on the container and have fun with your new try-on color.

Ready to Plunge

Now that you have gotten a taste of what color can and can't do for you with a temporary rinse, you might be ready to plunge ahead with something more permanent. Most of the colorings specially marked ''For Men Only'' don't contain peroxide and I would certainly never recommend one that does. No-peroxide colors may be used as often as needed, without going red in the sun or getting a harsh, dyed look. Remember that your temporary rinse just washes out, but semi-permanent colors do not wash out but will fade slightly as they grow out. Therefore you will need new applications every five or six weeks. By studying my chart you should have the correct idea of what the new color will do.

> RENN HINT: **Never try to color your very gray hair dark brown or black. Remember: gray is light around your face, and a much darker color will be harsh and will show twice as quickly when it starts growing in.**

If your natural hair is dark to medium-brown and you want to cover the gray, use a medium-warm brown. If your hair is lighter, a light-brown shade should be used, and if you don't want to cover the gray hairs completely, but want them to look like highlights instead, use a blond or sandy-color semi-permanent no-peroxide tint.

> RENN HINT: **With this method of going from a temporary rinse to a more lasting color using a semi-permanent tint, there is no big overnight change. You won't shock the folks at the office, since the color will look natural.**

A perfect time to change your hair color is during a vacation. You leave pale and gray, and then arrive back to work all suntanned and much younger-looking with no gray hair. I am certainly not down on gray hair—some men do look smashing —but as I said before, it is the way you feel that makes you love it or hate it.

RENN HINT: For a more natural look, especially if your natural hair color is toward the dark side, keep a little gray at the temples. This will also present a more dramatic and distinguished you.

Here's How You Do It

Before coloring, section off about an inch of hair all around your hairline. The parting should be slightly staggered so that when the hairline, or the part of the temple hair not being colored, is combed back and over the new color, there will be no line where one starts and the other stops. With long hair this is never a problem, but extra-short hair will be more

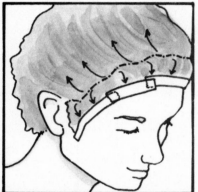

Section off small amount of hair in front to keep a little gray, and tape to forehead.

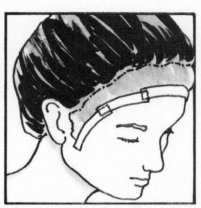

Apply color to rest of hair to color gray.

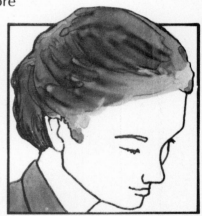

Natural-looking results.

difficult to do. After sectioning the hairline, comb it forward, and if it's short, you can Scotch-tape it to your cheek and forehead. Then apply the tint to the rest of the hair, taking special care *not* to get the color on the hair that you have combed forward. Follow the directions about the processing time and rinse all the color out before combing back the hairline section. An added dividend here is that since the hairline is still natural and untinted, the roots will not show as the color grows out, so the new color actually lasts twice as long.

   To Lighten Hair   Rinses and no-peroxide tints can cover gray and work a lot of different ways, but they cannot lighten hair. It takes peroxide mixed with a permanent tint or with a lightening mixture to lighten the hair.

   If your hair was once blonder in the summer than in the winter, there is no reason why you can't have that look again and have it be just as natural-looking.

For this lightening effect I think that my highlighting method, by customizing a frosting kit for home use, will work best, because it enables you to add a few highlights—or many highlights, whichever you want—all with the same kit. Though you may be willing to pay for quality, you can get a super bargain for around five dollars.

> RENN HINT: Follow all the tips and instructions in Chapter 4 and do light up your life. Highlights for men are best when they are done in connection with the sun, so that you can benefit from the combination of a tan with the lighter hair. They just seem to go together, giving you a more natural look.

For too-bright redheads with pink complexions Little boys with carrot-tops and freckles are cute when they are small, but if the color of your hair is still bright-orange at twenty-five, and the freckles have blended into a ruddy-pink skin tone, nothing could be worse. A medium- or light-brown no-peroxide tint over this red hair will give a strong and more masculine look to your skin and hair. The hair will be a softer tan-brown color, and the pink cast to the skin will look as if you've been to the beach rather than in a sauna. Now your hair color and the skin tone will complement each other rather than clash.

To Color a Mustache I have often suggested to men that they grow a mustache to hide a thin top lip or some other problem, only to laugh a few weeks later when I see their new proud growth a totally different color from their hair. They would surely have shaved it off, until I suggested changing the color! A medium-brown or dark-brown color, no-peroxide, can be used at home every few weeks without fear of risking that growing-out look. Color application is made easier by using a small artist's brush or special hair-color brush sold in drugstores. Protect the skin around the mustache with a little cold cream, to prevent any stains.

> RENN HINT: It is really amazing how strong and with-it a man can look with the right mustache or beard. Get a special small pair of scissors to keep your facial hair looking neat and perfect at all times.

Hairpieces It is not easy to find a good toupee. But if wear one you must, then make sure it's perfect. Don't buy one that has too much hair. Everyone's hair thins as he gets older, so remember that. Make sure the color matches yours, too. Though the cut is important, it's the color that counts most! As you get older, add highlights or a few gray hairs. These can be sewn in to match your own hair. Even if your hairpiece is old, it can be freshened up with a quick color treatment with a no-peroxide tint, and can be made a shade darker if your own color has changed. Just remember that dark, solid colors are not natural-looking, but shadings of slightly lighter tones look better as we get older.

Silver or That Beautiful Gray Hair I see men everywhere who must have beautiful gray hair that is hidden under a dull slate-colored rinse. Temporary rinses, after long and repeated use on gray and white hair, build up on the hair and stain it, taking away the natural shine and making the hair look artificial. If this is your problem, I suggest a home or salon hot-oil treatment that will lift out the old drab stain and give your hair new shine and sparkle. Maybe you won't have to recolor your hair after the treatment, but if you do, use a no-peroxide silver shade just to get rid of any yellow that might be present.

I think there is nothing more flattering to a man than a suntan and beautiful silver hair, but if it bothers you and makes you look and feel older, then by all means color it.

Let Me Introduce You to Some of My Clients

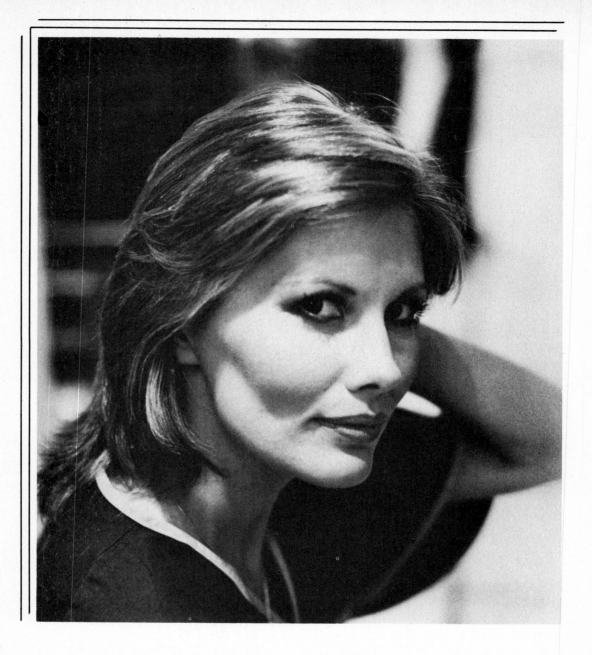

Maud Adams

One of the most beautiful women in the world—and certainly one of the nicest—Maud came to the States about twelve years ago, after winning a model contest in Sweden. She became an instant success, and her face has been on the cover of almost every major fashion magazine. She also has several films to her credit and is currently pursuing her movie career.

When Maud first came to me, her hair really needed help. It was suffering from overwork: too much bleach and not enough conditioning. I added depth and contrast by reverse streaking, while highlighting the new growth.

PHOTO CREDIT: ROBERT RENN

When I went to Paris to model I started streaking my hair. That was not the kind of fine streaking that you do now; my hair was almost orange then—awful. But I think that makeup was not as subtle then; it was the time of Jean Shrimpton and Twiggy and false eyelashes. We used to wear two or three pairs of eyelashes—that's the kind of makeup we used to wear—and your hair as well as your makeup had to be very dramatic.

You started doing my hair when I first came to New York, and in order to get away from the solid blond look which I'd ended up with, you first reverse-streaked my hair, but still kept it quite light. People expected me to be very blond, because I am Swedish, but you made me a newer, more natural blonde. Now I want my hair to look as if I don't do anything—very natural and blended in perfectly.

Sure, I'm tall and thin and have good cheekbones, which are basic requirements for a model, but I need to give nature a little help. I'm a pale, Northern type, so I need help with color on my cheeks and on my eyes. I don't like to wear a lot of makeup, just enough to give me a little color, and I do the same thing with my hair.

Psychologically this color gives one a little lift, a little emotional brightening up. Changing one's hair color, or giving it a lift with just highlights, is one of the best boosters I know.

A woman who is intelligent and secure within herself knows how important projecting a good image is. It affects her psychologically, as well as the people around her. I think that the most successful career women have spent time on their looks, on doing something that they know is complimentary to themselves. One learns over the years what suits one best and to choose wisely.

I think that this has to do with the security I feel; I can relax because now what I concentrate on is keeping myself and my hair in good condition. My new color is the most important step in this plan. Nature does not always give us the best, so why not help her a little!

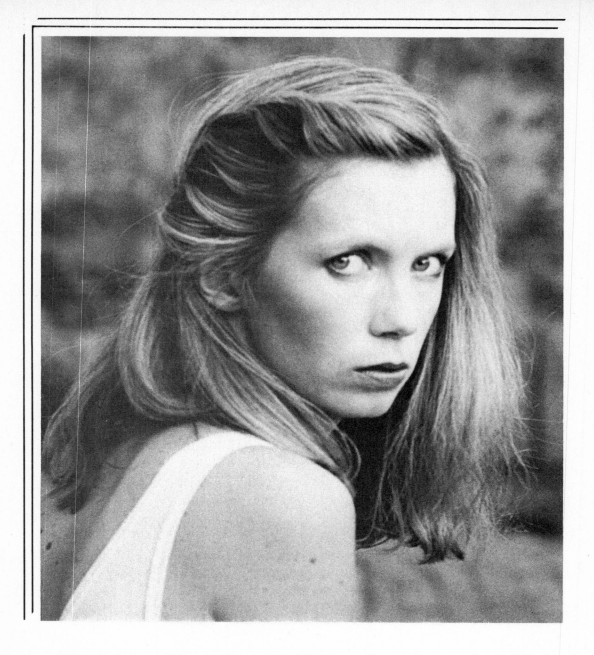

Mary Randolph Carter Berg

Attractive and down-to-earth, with a wonderful flair for finding the unusual, putting it together beautifully in an unexpected way, and always coming up with her own incredible style. Former beauty editor of *Mademoiselle* magazine, contributing editor on beauty and fashion for *New York* magazine, she is now creative director of Living Styles for the new Condé Nast publication, *Self.*

Carter's hair had been lightened with a one-process hair color, which gradually oxidized and turned brassy in the sun. We had been friends for several years before she actually turned to me for help, but when I finally got my hands on her, I simply added highlights every few months, giving her an overall blond look, but relieving her of the chore of monthly touch-ups.

PHOTO CREDIT: ARTHUR ELGART COURTESY CONDE NAST

first started to color my hair my sixteenth summer. I think it was the first time I'd really been in love, so maybe I was more aware of the way I looked. I got some Light and Bright and combed it in every time I went to the beach. My hair never seemed blond enough, so I kept combing in more and more each day and thought that it was absolutely beautiful. I saw some pictures of myself that summer and my hair was bright orange. The next stage was a shampoo-in color, sort of an ash blond, which I kept up at home until I met you.

I came to you because I wanted to free myself from the color I had ended up with and from the time I spent trying to keep up with it. My hair had gotten to be all one solid blond color, and the roots were just another solid color. I had to touch up about once a month or so. Since I don't have much time, I'm willing to devote more money; it's worth it.

If I didn't color my hair, it would be some sort of a drab brown or dirty blond, and that color does nothing for me. Once a little color came into my hair, it seemed to help my skin, everything . . . the smallest amount of color gives me a total lift.

My whole thing about hair color is very psychological, as it is for many people. A person may be depressed, and one of the things she can do immediately to change her life is to change her hair color. Just the psychological lift she gets from her brighter hair is enough to give her a whole new outlook on life.

If my hair looks great, I find I don't have to worry so much about other things. I wear a minimal amount of makeup, and I know that when my hair is done, the color enhances my complexion so much that I don't have to think about makeup. When I was one solid color all over, this was something I had to worry about because it washed me out so badly.

I've also found that ever since you've been doing my hair, the quality of it has improved. Now I have so much body because the color you've added has in turn given my hair more texture.

I love being a blonde . . . this natural kind of blonde. Whenever I toy with the idea of going back to my natural color, I let it go for a while and then I pull it all back, take a look and say absolutely not.

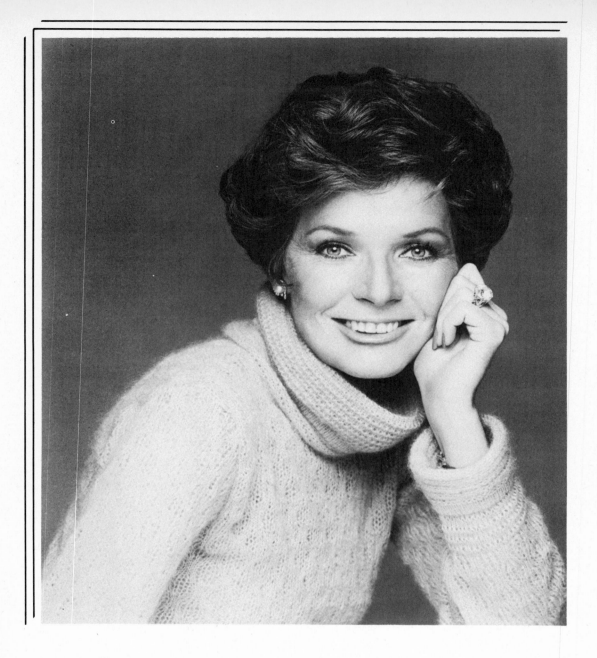

Polly Bergen

Talented actress, beauty and fashion consultant, author and a lady who knows what really works for her. She's vivacious and great fun, and everyone in the salon—staff and clients—love her visits.

For the last few years Polly had been covering up her gray with Loving Care, because she didn't want to dye her hair. But she found that the color wasn't lasting long enough for her fast-paced life between New York and California.

I added darker-brown streaks throughout the hair, and at the same time covered the gray strands with a more permanent no-peroxide color, giving her a low-maintenance program but the look of highlighted hair.

PHOTO CREDIT: FRANCESCO SCAVULLO

I think the very first time I colored my hair was when I was about fifteen and a friend put red henna on it. It stayed very purple-red for a very long time. The next time was when I was eighteen and was about to do a movie. They decided that I would make a great redhead. Oddly enough, I had been born a redhead, but my hair had gotten darker as I had gotten older, so I became a strawberry blonde. It was exactly the color of Rita Hayworth's hair, so I ended up using her hairpieces. I remember opening at the Maisonette in New York and the reviews started out, "The apricot-thatched Polly Bergen . . ." —whatever that means. The blond-red hair looked very natural with my pink-white skin, my freckles and my blue eyes, so when for another film my hair had to be dyed dark brown, people were horrified that I would allow my "natural" red hair to be covered up. I felt like a redhead, but I liked what the dark-brown hair did for my pale skin, so I stayed that way for about five or six years, until that turned out to be the color my hair had actually become.

Then one day, depressed about a personal relationship, I had my hair dyed back to the old red. But my skin had changed and had lost a lot of the natural color which had made the red work, and I had to wear a lot more makeup because I looked so washed out. I got tired of having to make up like a chorus girl all the time, so I decided to let my natural hair color grow in, only to find out that at the old age of about thirty, I had become about three-quarters gray. So I started dyeing it again, using a rinse, because it was quick and I could do it myself. The only problem with the rinse was that it faded, and since my hair is trimmed every week and cut every three weeks, I couldn't keep up with it. The first time I really found a correction for all of these problems was when I found you, and you began to highlight my hair.

As I get older, I've discovered that dark hair gives me a very hard look. My hair looks much better a little lighter, and your highlighting is perfect. I've discovered that I can go a lot longer without having my hair done and still have enough color so that I don't get washed out. Hair coloring to me is as important as putting on makeup; I could not do without either.

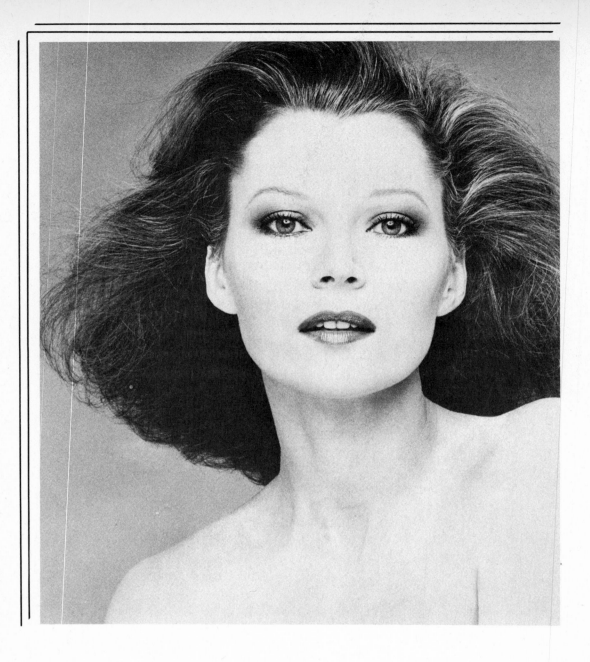

Audrey Butvay

A delicate but definite beauty, the epitome of New York chic, with a
fantastic beauty sense that works for her in her job as director of advertising
and creative services for an international cosmetic firm.

Audrey came to me with much darker hair, not feeling as if she
needed a color change, but wanting more of a "lift." I started adding subtle
highlights, gradually making her hair lighter, ending up with an overall
warmer effect.

PHOTO CREDIT: LES GOLDBERG

To be perfectly honest, I'd always thought that my own hair color was very pretty, and I like the natural look in women anyway. Then I heard about your work from one of our models. She had such exquisite hair, the highlights were so beautiful, that I could hardly tell with my critical eye whether it was natural or not. I wanted to have hair like that!

Over the years, as you've made my hair lighter, I've had to change my overall makeup. It's changed to go along with the hair color. I feel blonde now, and before I was definitely more brownette. My coloring, my makeup, the clothes I wear all go along with this new perception.

I think hair definitely has a lot to do with sexual appeal, with the whole look. That whole crowning-glory mystique is so true. If a woman's hair is shining, if it's special, if it's done right and the color is beautiful, that's what is attractive. I really don't think that a man will spot a blonde rather than a beautiful redhead or an incredible brunette. If a woman has the color that suits her best, a man will notice. *Do* blondes have more fun . . . I have fun all the time, blonde, brunette, streaked or unstreaked.

When your hair is shinier, prettier and you've got those highlights going, and you know it and you feel it, maybe you do have more fun. It helps you to have that extra bit of confidence. It's all very psychological. Two little streaks and see what they do . . . or three hundred streaks and a whole new you.

Getting hair color that lasts and looks right, that's what today's woman wants. My hair color is so natural and works so well for me that having it done four times a year is a small price to pay, literally, in both time and money, to look better and to feel free.

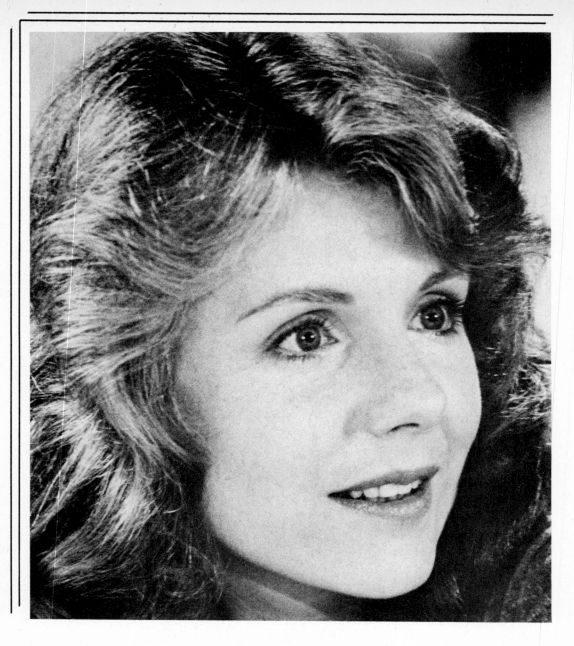

Jill Clayburgh

A delightfully charming and funny person with natural good looks, truly a new star of the seventies. She won the "best actress" award at the Cannes Film Festival for her starring role in *An Unmarried Woman.*

After filming *Gable and Lombard,* Jill's hair was a disaster area, and I had been recommended to give her hair a more believable darker-blond color instead of the all-over bleached blond she'd ended up with.

I alternated layers of dark blond with the lighter blond, which gave her hair a more textured, natural look. It has taken me at least two years to get Jill's hair back into condition, which was perfect timing for her new film *La Luna,* in which she had to become blond again.

PHOTO CREDIT: COURTESY TWENTIETH-CENTURY FOX

My mother always said that my hair was my worst feature, so I spent most of my time trying to ignore it. But then I saw myself on film and felt that it really looked too dark. I felt that the dark color dragged my face down. I tried streaks. They were wonderful, but I didn't keep them up.

Then the director of *Gable and Lombard* asked me to test, and they stuck this ghastly platinum wig on my head. Oh my God, when I think of that wig. I did the first test wearing it, but I looked like a drag queen. So they sent me off to have my hair bleached. It looked wonderful the first day; I was incredibly beautiful. Of course my scalp had huge welts all over it from sitting for so long with bleach on my head, but the color was beautiful. As the months went on it looked worse and worse, until finally by the end of the movie it looked as if I had tinsel falling out of my head. No one had told me that my hair was going to disintegrate. I suppose I did feel glamorous at first, but all too soon the problems started. All those touch-ups—it's like five o'clock shadow.

By the time I was finished with the film, I had to wear a wig over the blond hair to do a television show, because I was scared to death to have anyone out there touch my hair.

I did finally get another brown color to cover up the blond, and then my hair started to fall out. I never thought I'd have my own hair back until you came along. You saw it three degrees after its worst.

Now that my hair is highlighted, I feel like more of a natural blonde, an elegant blonde, not that awful hooker blonde. This way, it's not only more becoming to my pinkish, sometimes freckled skin, but it's easier. I'm lucky that I wash my face or brush my teeth when I'm not filming and I try to leave my hair alone as well; it gets so much abuse all day when I'm filming. Now the way my hair coloring is, I can always get it fixed up at the last minute before starting a film. It has proved to be both easier and more becoming. I love it.

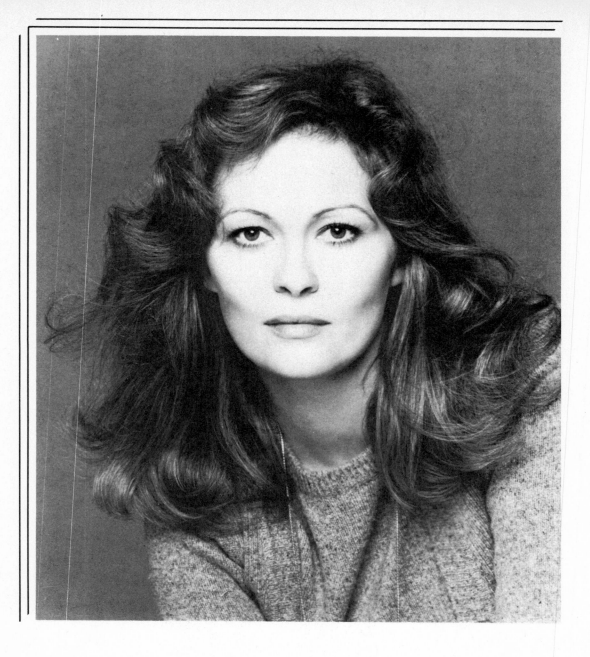

Faye Dunaway

A very natural, handsome woman with incredible bone structure, who is an exceptionally fine actress, renowned for her portrayals of many varied characters, such as her Oscar-winning performance in *Network*.

For the part of Laura Mars the studio thought that Faye should have red hair. Faye was totally against using the harsh chemicals that would have been required in order to make her hair that red, so the studio started experimenting on her with natural hennas. The result was harsh, blotchy and very unattractive.

I was called in to correct the henna mistakes and to create a new color for the part. I did this using no-peroxide colors, pleasing Faye, and we sustained the desired color throughout the filming.

PHOTO CREDIT: FRANCESCO SCAVULLO

think hair coloring is a more complicated thing for an actress than for the average woman. It's not simply a matter of changing from brunette to blonde or redhead. For just as each role contains its mystery of who the character is, it also holds the mystery of what the character must look like. The color of an actress's hair is almost as important as what clothes she wears, how she moves and the way she says her lines.

An actress changes her appearance with each role, and often this includes changing the color of her hair. Most film roles demand only a slight change, perhaps some streaking or highlighting for the camera to pick up. But I can think of two parts where the change was quite drastic. Bonnie, of *Bonnie and Clyde,* had to be that very light blonde. And Laura, of *Eyes of Laura Mars,* had to be a redhead. Obviously, wigs are a possibility. But wigs, even the best of them, are constricting. Imagine the difference between running one's fingers through a wig and doing the same thing with one's own hair. One is a careful gesture, the other is free.

Hair is indeed the crowning glory to one's identity. The transformation to another look, part of becoming another character, has its perils. In the usual coloring process hair often breaks and can be badly damaged. It happened to me after *Bonnie and Clyde.* Also, in every movie the usual ten or twelve weeks of filming are hazardous—a crash process as far as hair is concerned. In addition to the color processing, there is the constant touching up and settings, the rollers and dryers, and the hours under the hot lights of a film set.

What I found unique about you, Robert, was your concern for the health of my hair and your method of working. We discussed in detail the transformation you would create for the character I was going to portray as I saw her. You outlined every step of the process, discussing with me what was wrong and how you would correct it. I felt secure with your careful attention to each detail.

My own look is a free, natural one. That is what I feel happiest with. Between films I give my hair its needed rest, using only organic shampoo and conditioner and rarely setting it. When it is time to be a different person for a new film— someone perhaps with an entirely different hair color because the character demands it—then I have to come to you again for your skill and alchemy. Then, and most important to me, when the filming is over, you bring me back to the natural me.

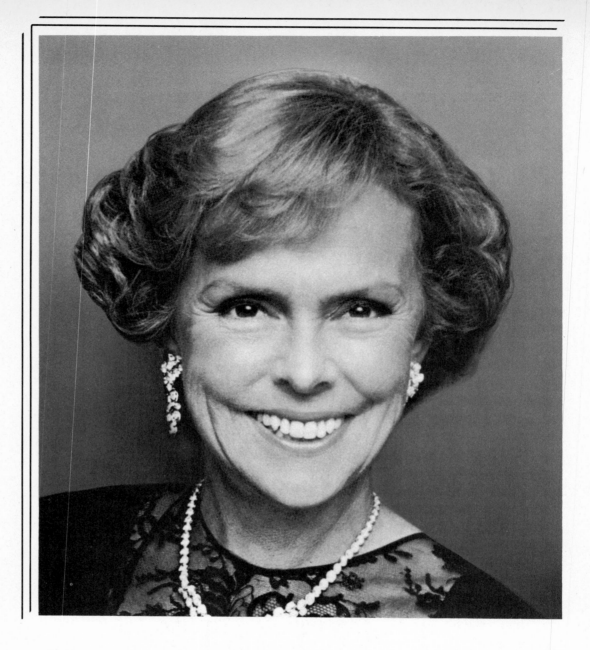

Eileen Ford

First lady of the modeling business and a beauty in her own right. She and her husband Jerry started the now world famous Ford Agency. Eileen with her direct, straightforward manner has an innate sense of what true beauty really is and has proven this by having discovered most of the great beauties of our time.

Eileen was facing that very common problem—the first appearance of gray. Definitely not a blonde type, Eileen has found that through the years, lighter hair is much more flattering. So instead of completely covering her gray hair, we use a lighter-color tint that plays up the gray hairs as lighter highlights.

PHOTO CREDIT: JAMES MOORE

The sight of my first gray hair started my thinking about coloring my hair. I began with one-process color, which is what I still use. I used the same tint as my natural color, but it became increasingly more difficult, because my hair is very dark brown and it was difficult to cover the gray.

Then I found that stuff you spray on to give you highlights. With that I had varying degrees of success, from sensational to catastrophic. Doing highlights at home was easier because I didn't want a frosted look, but in the end I had orange hair! You can only do so much for yourself.

I can't afford to have gray hair; I can't possibly write a book on "How to Look Younger," and lecture on the same topic with gray hair. You just don't look younger with gray hair: even if it's striking, you still look older. However, since one's skin gets paler as one gets older, very dark hair is too much of a harsh contrast. That's why highlighting is so perfect. It picks up dark hair, gives it pizzazz and vitality. Since hair photographs very dark compared with what it actually is, hair coloring is very important in the modeling business.

Hair coloring has been a tremendous force in this business. Obviously, our models make money doing hair-color ads, but if we couldn't lighten the hair, we would never have the same degree of success. To the average American an average American is blond and blue-eyed, and he doesn't recognize the fact that most of us have to get there chemically. Therefore, yes, blondes get more work . . . maybe they even have more fun.

However, it's the subtle hair coloring I'm talking about. Jerry didn't even notice that I'd had my hair colored the first three days, but people do react in a very positive way to how I'm looking and that makes me feel better. Sure, hair coloring is as important for me as it is for my models.

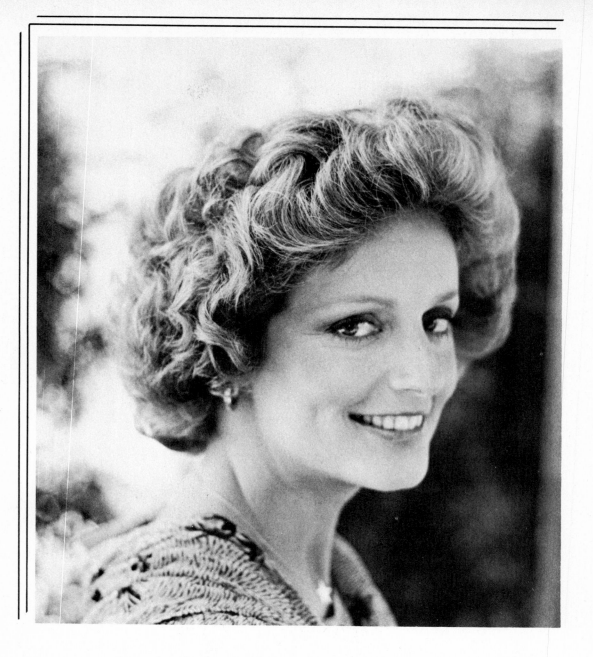

PHOTO CREDIT: ROBERT RENN

Sunny Griffin

Vivacious, talkative and beautiful. A top model since graduation from
college (with a degree in chemistry), Sunny can smile and sell you anything.
She is now Beauty and Fashion director for Avon Products, Inc. Who says
it's impossible to be a wife, a mother and a businesswoman?

Sunny's hair was very weird when I first saw her. It was long, the top
or crown area was brassy blond, and the rest of it was brown. To blend
this masterpiece together, I added blond highlights to the brown parts and
shadings of darker brown on the top. It was a lot of work.

I have this picture in my head of being in college with all the girls lined up at sinks in the bathroom, pouring bleach on our heads, everybody coming out orange. This was about 1959, right in the age of "Is it true blondes have more fun?"

Hair coloring has been extraordinarily important to me because it's been so much of my image. I've always felt drab with darker hair, and I feel that with the name "Sunny" one has a certain obligation to remain blond. I have far from perfect features, so much of my look depends on my hair, on the color and the shape of it . . . how it makes my face work.

I think that if your hair looks terrific you do, and the reverse is true. The shine, the texture and the shape of your hair are all important, which is to say that the color is just as important, because of what it does for your face. Drab hair drains the color out of my face. I have very fair but very sallow skin, and my hair is naturally dishwater. Put this pale-yellow skin with dishwater hair, and it looks really revolting. So putting sunlighting into my hair (which is what I consider you do to my hair) really adds sparkle to my face. I remember that my hair was striped when I first came to you, and you did something for each level of stripes, so that in the end it all had this wonderful natural look.

I'm proud as heck of my hair. To have people look at it and think it looks natural is a tremendous compliment to you as well as to me. After it's done I notice how much brighter it all is, and even more important, how it cheers me up. When my hair's drab, I feel drab, but when it's all full of sunlights, I feel . . . dare I say it? . . . sunny.

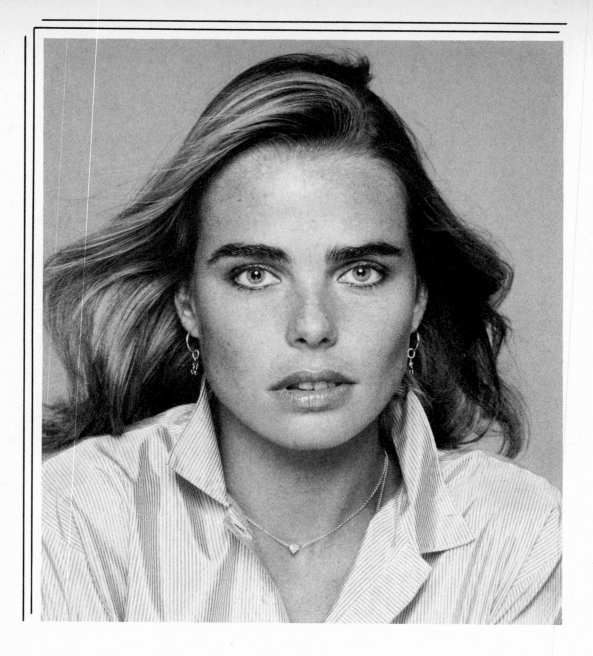

Margaux Hemingway

Striking example of all-American good looks, with her own personal style, Margaux, granddaughter of Ernest Hemingway, has quickly become famous in her own right. Her face is known all over the world as the million-dollar "Babe" for Fabergé, and she is an up-and-coming actress.

Margaux's hair was in terrible shape when I first saw her. It suffered from a combination of chemicals and too much sun. I had to both correct the color and have her hair literally "picture perfect" by the next day for the start of the filming of *Lipstick*. It was some job!

PHOTO CREDIT: P. RATAZZI

The first time I colored my hair was about a year and a half before I met you. My hair is light brown, almost blond, and was naturally much lighter in the summer than in the winter. However, when I was on a fishing trip off the tip of the Baja Peninsula, I started putting lemon juice on my hair, and in that strong sun it really turned blond. Then I started using Sun-In at the beach, because I loved being so much blonder than usual. When I did the first advertising campaign for Fabergé's "Babe" that was the color of my hair.

But, between the sun and chlorine, my hair was beginning to look green. That's when Francesco Scavullo brought you out to California to fix my hair for *Lipstick*. They still wanted it to be blond, but a more elegant, shaded blond. You streaked it with several darker shades, and at first I freaked out because it looked darker, but then I saw it on film and it still looked very light. It was darker, but at the same time it was more my natural color. It really worked well.

The whole idea of a new hair color actually helped me in my role for the film, since I was now different from that blond Fabergé model. The new color was much more sophisticated, because it was much more textured, the way hair is naturally. When the camera is moving, it sees everything, so you want every single hair in place. When you arrived on the scene, that was just one less thing to worry about. That is the beauty of going to an expert. I know that my new hair color makes me feel better and frees me to think about my work. Now I know how good my hair can look, having worked with an expert like you.

I love being a blonde. The only times I've been upset about color was when I wasn't. Once I put a temporary rinse on my hair for a ski race. It made my hair dark brown, which was sort of fun for a while, but it was much too severe. Another time, somebody bleached my eyebrows and they grew back orange. Touch my eyebrows, you're dead.

When I have a tan, either from the beach or from skiing, and I'm feeling good about my healthy, shining blond hair, I'm really feeling good about me.

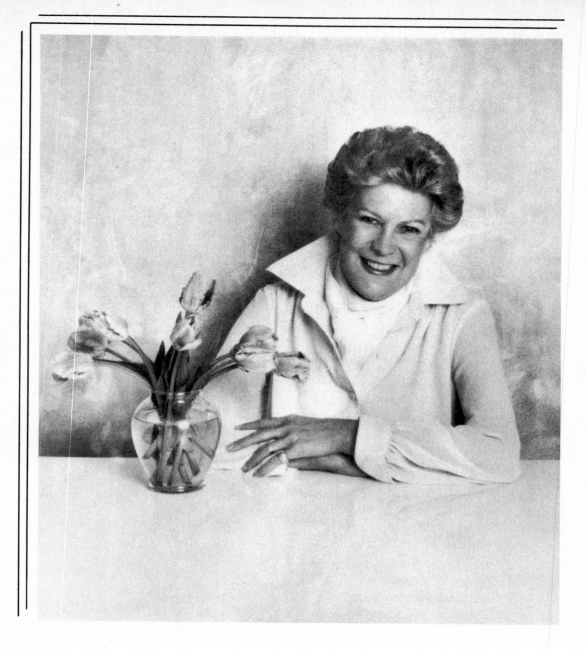

Sylvia Porter

A financial wizard, with healthy good looks and a charming wit. Author (her *The Money Book* was the number-one best seller in 1975, '76 and '77) as well as television personality, her column on finance and consumer economics appears in the New York *Daily News* and in over four hundred newspapers all over the country, and throughout the world.

Sylvia covered up her natural, beautiful silvery hair with dark-brown dye. This was not only harsh and unbecoming, but the dye tended to gradually oxidize and turn red. I added lots of blond highlights to complement the silver growing in and covered the old, fading tint with a no-peroxide light-brown color to soften the growing-out stage.

PHOTO CREDIT: ALEX GOTFRYD

A friend of mine, a TV producer, walked in one day with the most wonderful highlighting, which you had done for her. She said that my hair really looked too dark for me, so off I went to you to get something done to my dark but aging hair. You didn't say what I should or should not do but started right in working on me, and the results were a miracle . . . a complete transformation. You took it from dark and dull and unbecoming hair to a light, brighter shade, which not only brightened up my face, but which significantly brightened up my whole outlook on myself and on my whole life at that time. I had been going through a traumatic personal experience and this color change gave me a lift, which is very difficult to explain. I think when these personal traumas come along one needs a change—from the ultimate, a facelift, to the intermediate step of changing the color of one's hair. This change can be an indescribable benefit to you and for your spirits. I felt that this change for me came at a time that was crucial in my life, and I shall forever be grateful.

You highlighted my hair, which added just enough blond to lighten up and brighten up my skin, which is quite olive. I think it added youthfulness as well as gaiety to my face, and no matter whether it did or didn't, I certainly think it does— and that's what is important. And what's more important is that I thought so first, and then the complements came pouring in. I had my pictures in the newspapers across the country changed, and as a result I got a lot of letters. The people who work with me were saying "Hey, you look great, what have you done?" I think that you've done me a service that would be hard to translate into money, but (I want to add, by the way, that your prices are outrageous) it was worth it. I always have to justify to myself what I spend— after all, it is my profession. I have convinced myself that I have more than offset the cost of the color treatments, because I just don't need to have my hair colored as often. I've even learned to blow it dry myself, because it was cut short the same time as it was highlighted, so now I am free to go away for more than a month without worrying about my hair at all. I travel a lot and this makes a huge difference. I feel free and wonderful.

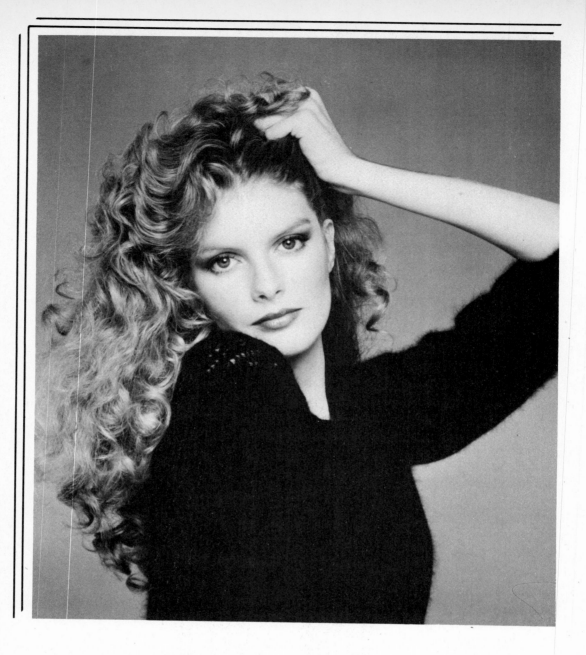

Rene Russo

The beautiful model on my cover was sent to me by famous photographer Francesco Scavullo. When you see Rene for the first time you realize why she is much sought after for magazine layouts, covers and television work. Living in California and practically commuting to New York keeps Rene on the move. Her shy wit and vulnerability make one want to care for her. Rene has the most incredible hair of any model I've worked with, thick with just the right amount of natural curl for lots of body. The only thing her hair needed was to be made blonder so that it would photograph better.

PHOTO CREDIT: FRANCESCO SCAVULLO

The first time I colored my hair was with you, and it was incredible. I loved it so much. Your blonder color helped me because I think that I look better blond and blond models seem to work more in this country. I think I have very pronounced features and that blond hair softens them; with dark hair I seem to look too severe. I love girls with dark hair . . . I think it's so sexy. If I could have been born with any color hair, my choice would be black hair with that wonderful white skin and blue eyes. My skin tone would have to go with the dark hair. I mean I wouldn't just dye my hair black . . . it would look terrible. You have to have the face, and I don't have that kind of skin; mine is ruddy. But my new blond complements my ruddy complexion and I like to look more baby . . . more round face, which I feel softens my pronounced features.

Someone on the coast talked me into getting a perm, and what would normally work on natural hair was a disaster for me. Luckily, I have very strong hair, but because my hair is so long I had to live with that permanent for over a year. The only thing that saved my hair during that year was constant conditioning and a layered cut. I realize now how difficult it is to have a perm on very blond hair, particularly on very long, very blond hair. If I had to do it all over again, I would definitely get an okay from you, or better yet, I'd ask you to do it. If you refused, I wouldn't have a perm at all, because I trust your judgment. Now I condition my hair every single day, since that's how often I have to wash it because of my work. A lot of people don't realize that if you color your hair, you have to condition it accordingly.

Sometimes I use neutral henna on my hair. It doesn't really help the condition of my hair, but it does make it feel a bit thicker. I was curious though, as to why, when I'd used the henna, my conditioner didn't seem to work as well, until you told me that the henna coats the hair shaft, so the conditioner literally *can't* penetrate the hair. It just goes to show how much we don't know about hair. A model's hair is everything . . . it can get her a job or lose one for her, and I'm not going to take any more chances.

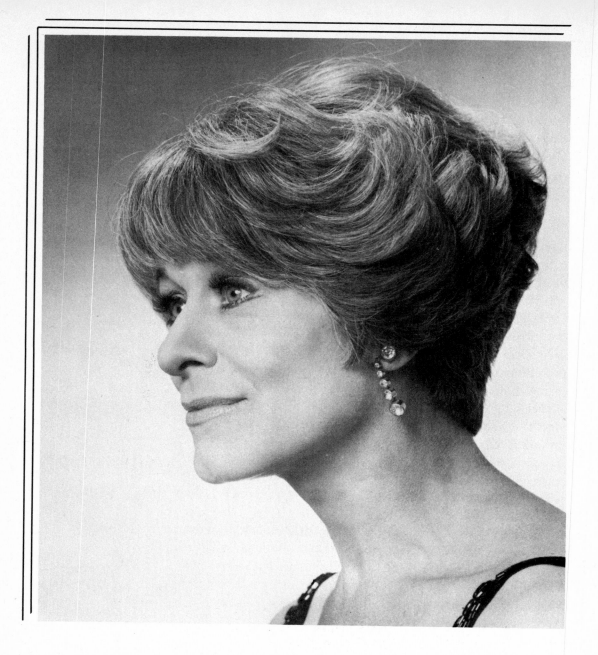

Gretchen Wyler

Singing and dancing star of Broadway and television, Gretchen is a twenty-four-hour worker for her many projects, including her own Animal Shelter in upstate New York. Full of good looks and boundless energy, she is constantly sought after for television appearances, concert series and for her lectures on animal rights. When Gretchen came to me she was sort of half-grown-out blond with her natural light brown coming in. She was finally ready for a more natural look.

PHOTO CREDIT: KEN DUNCAN

I was always known as that big bleached blonde from *Silk Stockings* on Broadway. In the fifties and sixties I was absolutely solid blond. Of course in those days it was more fashionable to be blond, but today it's an outrage. I cringe when I see people who are not hip enough to know that look is very out, and that the color of hair, in order to be really chic and beautiful, should never be solid anything.

I made my hair-color change for professional reasons, but it was one of the most important moves I've ever made. When I came to stand by for Lauren Bacall in *Applause,* the producer of the show asked me if I would mind making my hair a different color, as it would look all wrong if I had to go on for Bacall. At that point I hadn't seen my real color since I was eighteen, when I had gone really blond for *Guys and Dolls.* So I dyed it a light brown to see what would grow in. It came in a combination of light brown and dark ash blond. Then I started coming to you, to get a little more life into it by highlighting it and making it a little more glamorous. I guess if it hadn't been for Lauren Bacall, I would still be walking around with bleached blond hair.

I'll never change my hair color again, because this is exactly right for me, the person, rather than the character I happen to be playing at the moment. I'm more comfortable without all that blond hair, to tell the truth, because I always had a hard time living up to that super-glamour image. I'm really a little more regular than all that.

For twenty years I never washed my own hair. I had to go to the hairdresser every week just to keep up with the color, so my hair had always been a hideously time-consuming and expensive problem. But now, with what we do—only about four times a year for the highlights—the upkeep is negligible.

I think that it takes a certain amount of courage to deal with a change in hair color, particularly when one has reached about fifty. Then, when everything has started to sag a little, hair is the one thing that can be easily controlled, with hair coloring. The only trouble is that the tendency is to try to keep young by keeping bright blond or bright red hair, and this is all wrong. Remember the saying that God gave us gray hair as we age to soften the fading skin and to soften our features, and the natural process can be made that much better by going to someone like you, someone who believes in you, in making the best of the best you've got.

In Conclusion

Now you know how important hair color is and how it can change your looks and the way you feel about yourself. Hair color can add sparkle, texture and body to your hair, but the success of color depends on how well it complements your skin tone (olive skin doesn't go with red hair) and on looking natural (brunettes should never become platinum blondes). You've got to face the reality!

You know about the various kinds of color and which one will fill your needs. If you follow the step-by-step easy color guide for doing it at home, you'll find you'll be able to achieve professional results without having to go to a beauty salon. If you feel you need a little professional reinforcement, you know what to ask for.

You know, too, how to correct even the most disastrous color mistakes without risk of more damage to the hair—by using *no-peroxide* colors, which will work on damaged hair or over hair that is stained with henna, and which will last as long as other hair dyes that contain peroxide.

Remember, the color of your hair is only as good as the condition—healthy hair is what makes your color work. With a minimum of products, you can rebuild damaged hair, put body and shine back into sun-dried hair, or simply maintain your healthy hair at home.

Hair color is a fact of life, and just about everybody is concerned about the proper color. I hear from people all over the country about their hair problems and I've discovered that though the people may be different, the problems are the same. You've probably discovered that at least one of the celebrities in this book has a hair-coloring need similar to your own. There is no reason why you should not have the same answers to your hair-coloring problems as those I give every day in the salon, and there is no reason why you too should not be able to discover the incredible difference that hair color can make in your life.

Glossary of Terms

ACID—Chemical compound containing hydrogen ions that reacts to a base forming a salt; having a PH of less than 7.

ACID RINSE—A mixture of water and lemon juice or water and vinegar.

AERATION—Airing; giving a fluid more air.

ALKALINE—Having the properties of an alkali (hydroxide of a metal) with a PH of more than 7.

ALLERGIC—A sensitivity to certain substances, causing an unpleasant reaction.

ALLERGY TEST—A test to determine the existence or nonexistence of extreme sensitivity to certain foods or chemicals that do not usually affect most people. Sometimes referred to as predisposition test, patch test or skin test before application of a hair dye.

ASH—Drab; a shade in hair tinting that contains no red or gold tones.

ASH BLOND—A blond shade of hair that is not brassy.

BLEACHING SOLUTION—Used to remove or lighten hair color; usually 20-volume peroxide is mixed with ammonia or other commercial agents.

BLENDING—A merging of one tint with another.

BLONDING—Prelightening hair to get it ready for a toner.

BLOND ON BLOND—A combination of blond tones on one head of hair, usually one blond base color with highlights or streaks of a lighter blond.

BODY—Solidity or thick texture, in hair.

BODY PERMANENT—A permanent wave given to finer hair to impart texture and thickness without a visible wave or curl.

BRASSY TONE—A harsh, faded-quality hair color with gold or orange overtones.

BREAKAGE—A condition of hair that is broken and splitting as a result of excessive bleaching or chemicals.

BRITTLE HAIR—Dry, fragile hair that is easily broken.

COATING—Residue left on the hair shaft.

COLOR REMOVER—A product designed to remove dye from the hair; a dye solvent.

COLOR TEST—The process of washing or drying a strand of hair while coloring, to determine progress during tinting or bleaching.

COVERAGE—Having the color or tint take on gray or white hair.

COLOR-FAST—Usually a mild shampoo formulated for gentle cleansing and protecting the stability of the color of tinted hair.

COLOR FILLER—A preparation used to provide fill for porous spots in the hair during tinting, bleaching or permanent waving.

COLORIST—A qualified hairdresser and cosmetologist who is a specialist in hair coloring.

COLOR RINSE—A temporary rinse that gives a transparent coating of color to the hair.

COLOR SHAMPOO—A permanent hair dye that is formulated to apply all over the head, like a shampoo, to eliminate the sectioning and involved application of touch-ups. Usually mixed with equal parts of 20-volume peroxide.

COMPOUND HENNA—Egyptian henna to which has been added other dye preparations.

CORTEX—The largest and middle part of the hair structure.

CONDITIONER—Any product formulated for the reconstruction and care of the hair.

CONTRAST—A term in coloring used to compare the different tones that are easily distinguished from one another.

CROWN OF THE HEAD—The top back part of the head.

CUTICLE—The outside layer of the hair.

DAMAGED HAIR—A hair condition that results from overprocessing of chemicals.

DANDRUFF—A flaking of the scalp caused by excess dryness.

DANDRUFF SHAMPOO—A commercially prepared product that is used to control and eliminate dandruff when used as directed.

DENSE—Thick or heavy.

DENSITY—The number of hairs per square inch at the scalp.

DETERGENT—A synthetic soap.

DEVELOP—The processing time required for a tint or bleach to take effect.

DEVELOPER—20-volume peroxide mixed with tint or bleach to make it work.

DIMENSIONAL COLORING—Two or three shades of the same hair color used on the same head to give depth and shine.

DRAB—To add ash tones or to dull a brassy color down.

DYE—Any color product that will permanently change one's hair color.

DYE REMOVER—A product that is used to remove color stains from the hairline after tinting a dark color.

ELASTICITY—The ability of hair to be stretched and return to its original length.

FRAMING—Coloring just the hair around the face a shade or two lighter than the rest of the hair.

FADE—To disappear gradually.

FINE—A quality of hair where each hair is slender and smooth, not thick or coarse.

FROSTING—A process of bleaching tiny strands of hair all over the head with the aid of a plastic cap, followed by a toner on the bleached streaks.

FORMULA—Term used for the special proportions or mixture of products in coloring.

HAIR BLEACHING—Removing or lightening the natural color of hair.

HAIRLINE—The front edge of the scalp where the hair starts growing.

HAIRPIECE—A partial wig.

HAIR ROOT—The part of the hair that is below the surface of scalp.

HAIR SHAFT—The part of the hair which grows out of the scalp.

HAIR STRAIGHTENER—A special chemical product used to make kinky or very curly hair straight.

HAIR TINTING—The process of adding color pigment to the hair.

HALO LIGHTENING—Highlights on the crown section of hair only, usually a few shades lighter than the rest of the hair.

HARD WATER—Water containing certain salts of calcium or magnesium that do not allow soap to lather or rinse out.

HEATING CAP—An electrical insulated cap with different heat settings, used in scalp and hair treatments.

HIGH-FASHION BLONDING—The term from the sixties for a double-process bleach and toner.

HIGHLIGHTING—The introduction of slightly different shades to increase the brightness and shine of the hair.

HYDROGEN PEROXIDE—An oxidizing agent used to mix with hair dye and bleach to make them work properly.

ICING—Another term for the process of lightly frosting hair.

LIGHTENER—A chemical agent or bleach used to remove the color from the hair.

MARBLEIZING—A process in hair coloring: interweaving sections of lighter and darker colors within one head of hair.

MEDIUM HAIR—A texture of hair that is somewhere between fine and coarse.

MEDULLA—The innermost layer of the hair structure; or the center of the hair fiber.

MELANIN—The tiny grains in the cortex layer of the hair that determines the natural color of one's hair.

MESHE—The French term for streaking.

METALLIC DYES—Permanent dyes that contain metal salts.

MUTATION BLONDING—Blending lighter and darker shades of blond on a single head, blond on blond.

NEUTRAL—In chemistry, neither acid nor alkaline, having a PH of 7.

NEUTRAL BLOND—A color neither ash nor gold, usually a beige-blond.

NEUTRALIZER—The agent in straightening or permanent waving that stops the action of the cold-wave lotion.

ORGANIC—A substance derived from natural or live organisms.

OVERLAP—When tint or bleach is allowed to run on to previously colored hair, resulting in a different line of color or eventually hair damage.

OVERPOROSITY—A condition where hair reaches an undesirable state because of too many chemicals on the hair, expanding the hair shaft and making it like a sponge; very difficult to color or correct.

OXIDATION—The process in coloring that takes place after 20-volume peroxide is mixed with the dye or bleach to be used; the fading of peroxide tints because of sun or other chemicals, resulting in a brassy tone of hair.

PATCH TEST—A predisposition test used to tell if someone is allergic to a dye or color product.

PENETRATING COLOR—A hair dye or tint that is mixed with 20-volume peroxide and penetrates into the hair shaft to give permanent color change.

PH (POTENTIAL HYDROGEN)—The degree to which substance is acid or alkaline.

PRELIGHTEN—The first step in bleaching, which takes the color out of the hair, getting it ready to receive the toner or special shade of blond.

PROCESSING TIME—The period of time it takes to achieve the desired results in coloring hair.

PROGRESSIVE DYES—Hair-color restorers that get darker and darker with continued applications.

RETOUCH—Application of color or straightener only to the new growth of hair.

ROOTS—The growth of hair nearest the scalp where the natural hair color, different from the applied color, is growing in.

SALLOW—Skin tone with a yellowish cast.

SEMI-PERMANENT HAIR COLOR—Contains no peroxide and doesn't go into the hair shaft; it coats the outside layer and lasts for several weeks.

SINGLE PROCESS—A permanent hair tint or dye that is mixed with peroxide; colors and lightens at the same time. Sometimes referred to as the base color.

SOAP CAP—To add shampoo to the remaining tint mixture and work through the faded ends in the final step of a single-process touch-up.

STRAND TEST—To apply a small amount of color, or other substance to be used, on a small strip of hair to find out what the results will be before going ahead with the process.

STREAKING—The method of adding lighter strands throughout the hair.

SUNBURST—The method of adding natural golden streaks to the top surface of the hair to make it look as if it were done by the sun.

TEXTURE OF HAIR—The general quality as to the coarseness or fineness of the hair.

TINT—Permanent hair dye.

TIPPING—Making only the tips of the hair lighter.

TONE—The special color or hue; the process of adding the second step or blond coloring after the bleaching step in two-process blonding.

VIRGIN HAIR—Natural hair that has never been colored or subjected to any other chemical process.

Index